Forgive
and
Remember

Charles L. Bosk

Forgive and Remember

Managing Medical Failure

The University of
Chicago Press
Chicago and London

The University of Chicago Press, Chicago 60637
The University of Chicago Press, Ltd., London
© 1979 by the University of Chicago.
All rights reserved.
Published 1979
Paperback edition 1981
Printed in the United States of America
00 99 98 97 96 95 94 93 92 91   8 9 10 11 12

Library of Congress Cataloging in Publication Data

Bosk, Charles L.
  Forgive and remember.

  Bibliography: p.
  Includes index.
  1. Surgery—Study and teaching (Graduate)—Social
aspects.   2. Surgical errors.   3. Surgery—Quality control.
4. Surgeons.   5. Social control.   I. Title.
RD28.A1B67   617   78-16596
ISBN 0-226-06679-7
ISBN 0-226-06680-0 (paperback)

To the memory of my
mother and father,
whose norms I cherish,
whose quasi-norms I
miss

Contents

Acknowledgments

Field work, like surgery, is a "body-contact" sport, and the surgeons at Pacific Hospital never shrank from this contact. In what were often very trying circumstances, they were considerate, candid, and courteous beyond the limits of any social and academic obligation. If they taught me nothing else, the surgeons taught me that delivering high-quality humane care is hard work. This study is a testimony to their openness and honesty which the use of pseudonyms belies.

While the surgeons were teaching me that high-quality care is hard work, a number of sociologists were trying to teach me the same lesson about sociological research. This work is better for their support, encouragement, and criticism. Fred Strodtbeck introduced me to the problems with which this dissertation deals, and constantly challenged me to find ways for documenting the reliability and validity of my inferences. Charles Bidwell often saw more clearly than I what I was struggling to say, and was a useful guide through and disposer of needlessly labyrinthine arguments. I owe a singular debt to Barry Schwartz. His insistence that I look beyond the particulars of the field situation to more general social processes improved this work immeasurably. Odin Andersen provided both intellectual and financial assistance through National Center for Health Services Training Grant, HS 00080-08 through 12. Renée C. Fox read and extensively commented on various versions of this manuscript. Her colleagueship and support have been invaluable to me. I cannot do justice to her contribution to this work and to my own growth as a sociologist of medicine in a simple acknowledgment and/or appreciative footnote. Harold Bershady read and gently but firmly critiqued numerous drafts of the manuscript.

Marjorie Waxman, my wife, helped in ways too numerous to

recall. She provided support and encouragement during the very difficult first days of field research; she listened and asked searching questions as I began to develop my analyses; she extended my own thinking by drawing on her own stock of clinical experience; and she insisted that calling an unclear argument "sociological" does little to improve its clarity—her criticisms sent me back to the writing table more times than I like to remember. Were it not for her sense of humor and proportion I would never have finished this work.

A number of friends and associates also provided support, encouragement, and feedback. I am especially thankful to Bruce Atherton, Jarl Dyrud, Margaret Ensminger, Bill and Roseann Gallery, Joel Frader, Jeffrey Hantover, Paul Hirsch, Shepard Kellam, Sue Lelito, Victor Lidz, Jim Lynch, Ann Lyons, Samuel P. Martin III, Peter Meyer, Boyd Slomoff, and Judith Tribbett. The Guttman Foundation generously provided funds for the typing of this manuscript.

one

Introduction

At 6:30 A.M., only a few physicians and staff walk the still-darkened corridors of Pacific Hospital. Within an hour, the hospital will pulse with activity: nurses will wheel medication carts and chart racks down the halls; technicians will draw patients' blood, orderlies will place patients on line for the various diagnostic and therapeutic procedures the hospital provides; vendors will hawk the morning newspaper; and teams of physicians and students will make rounds on their patients. In the predawn, however, there is no hint of the burst of activity to come. A lone houseofficer trudges down the hall. A few nurses from the night shift gather at their station, chat while charting the previous night's activity, and share a last cup of coffee before ending their day at the beginning of everyone else's. Only one small group of physicians is already engaged in the purposive and feverish activity that one associates with the hospital during the day. For them, the day is in full swing. This group of physicians moves from bleary-eyed patient to bleary-eyed patient while jotting down what work must be done that day. Their movements are swift and precise; no energy is wasted in extraneous chatter with patients or each other.

Who are these few physicians? Why are they up so early? They are members of the surgical housestaff of Pacific Hospital. The two or three days a week on which the services they are assigned to operate, these men and women begin rounds at 6:00 A.M. so that they can be scrubbed, capped, gowned, and ready to operate on their first patient at precisely 8:00 A.M. This starting time is important to them for a number of reasons. First, they know if they miss it they will be behind schedule all day. Although the twenty-minute difference between 8:00 A.M. and 8:20 A.M. is not great, it is often the difference between a hurried lunch and a twelve-hour fast. Moreover, this is not a quiet, meditative fast, but one during which the hungry houseofficer must remain standing; assist with or perform operative procedures; pass "ad hoc" quizzes on anatomy and the advisability of various treatment modalities; engage in witty repartee with his superordinate, the attending surgeon; or accept silently his role as butt of his superior's jokes. Second, houseofficers who are not ready on schedule appear to their superordinates as inefficient, lazy, or unreliable. As houseofficers well know, "attendings" do not suffer wasted time—or those who force them to waste it—gladly. A houseofficer's good name rests in part on his ability to keep events running on schedule.

For eighteen months, I was a participant-observer of the surgical training program of Pacific Hospital. Three interrelated problems captured my interest and attracted me to this field setting. First was a question of social control. On precisely what kinds of behavior does a houseofficer's good name rest? What kinds of actions discredit him? How are evaluations of competence constructed by superiors, how are these evaluations shared, and how consequential are they? To use the vocabulary of Everett C. Hughes (1971), I was interested in how a segment of the medical profession exercises its "license" and "mandate."

Second was the question of social support. The superordinate's task is a delicate one. He must control mistakes. Yet at the same time, if he wishes to train competent, independent, and (eventually) autonomous professionals, he must allow his subordinates enough room to make the honest errors of the inexperienced. To allow this requires a certain cold-blooded calculation on the part of the superordinate. On the one hand, he needs to restrain himself from taking charge of situations too quickly lest he damage a subordinate's confidence. On the other hand, he needs to know when to rescue a subordinate—and patient—lest a surgical accident shake the novice's belief in his abilities. So the superordinate has a dual problem: (1) he must control his subordinate's performance and make sure that errors are corrected and not repeated, and (2) he must allow his subordinates room to make errors or they will never learn the judgments and techniques necessary to perform properly. At all times we should remember that this give-and-take between ranks is more than a mere academic exercise; the clinical material for these lessons is another human being who has placed his life in the surgeon's hands. Surgical superordinates who are permissive run the risk of abusing the patient's trust, while those who are restrictive may retard or destroy the careers of fledgling surgeons. The forces that lead a superordinate to monitor his subordinates' behavior more closely or those that lead him to forego close supervision are therefore not trivial matters. Because the consequences of these different modes of control and support are so fateful, rationales must be provided for their employment. Studying the different modes of control and their rationales will allow us to understand how a group of professionals conceptualizes its privileges and responsibilities.

Third was the question of sustaining individual commitments, motivation, and action in the face of failure. How does the surgeon cope with the knowledge that his clumsiness, forgetfulness, or tardiness contributed to another's death and/or suffering? How does the individual surgeon accept this responsibility and yet not shrink from future action? All groups possess devices for making failure a normal and accountable feature of everyday life. Surgeons are no different from the rest of us in this respect; the difference lies in the consequences of a failure. We assume that where the possibility of such consequential failure exists on each and every occasion for action, there will be powerful, shared devices for coping with these failures. Again, this is not a trivial matter, for to understand and analyze these devices is tantamount to analyzing the structure of the profession's conscience: its sense of right and wrong, and its sense of how large the gray area between them is.

This report centers on three themes: (1) How a professional group draws a boundary around itself and determines its own identity through the selection and rejection of recruits. (2) How superordinates attempt to control performance and how subordinates accept or avoid such controls in a professional training program. Of particular importance here is how norms of responsibility to patients and colleagues are articulated and how their violations are sanctioned. (3) How a professional copes with the existential problem of the limits of his skill and of his knowledge. In the course of things a surgeon's best efforts will sometimes fail and he must explain this failure to himself, his colleagues, and the family of his patient. We are interested in how the surgeon achieves accountability to each of these significant audiences and in what situations the surgeon fails to achieve this accountability. Taken together the three issues of membership in a professional group, social control of performance in that group, and shared patterns of explaining, understanding, and neutralizing failure and error are critical not only to our understanding of surgeons but indeed to all of the professions in modern American society.

These are, of course, not new issues; they have been much rehearsed in the sociology of medicine and the sociology of the professions. If these issues are not new, why engage them here? First, I want to recapture and refine the old Durkheimian insight that each occupational group possesses its own morality. I want to specify what for the surgeon is the "complex of ideas and sentiments, [the] ways of seeing and [of] feeling, [the] certain intellectual and moral framework distinctive of the entire group." As an occupational group, surgeons have a collective conscience. I shall make clear what it is, how it is formed, and what functions it serves. I then want to examine how this conscience serves the solidarity of the professional group and at what cost to the larger society. I want to know if any element in this "intellectual and moral framework" defines the essence of a profession in our society. Second, the occupational morality of the surgeon tells us much about how members of a profession interpret, act on, and defend their prerogative of social control. Any programmatic change which intends to make professionals more accountable to clients must of necessity start with a complex phenomenological understanding of what currently passes for accountability and how it is achieved. Field research such as this informs policy by grounding it in a firm understanding of how participants con-

struct their social worlds. It is only from this concrete understanding of the present, practical order that any changes in the
existing interactional politics of social control can be negotiated.

The Field Setting and
Data Collection

The setting for this study of how surgeons detect, categorize, and
sanction error is Pacific Hospital. Pacific Hospital is an elite
medical institution affiliated with a major medical school and
university. In both medicine and surgery, it has a luminous
reputation and a grand tradition. Everywhere one looks, one is
reminded of Pacific's special place in the medical universe.
Portraits of distinguished faculty grace hallways and classrooms.
Lecture rooms and entire wings of the hospital are named after
past greats that Pacific claims as its own. In addition, Pacific
sponsors several endowed lectures a year which are named for its
most eminent embodiments of the clinician-researcher ideal.
These lectures are given by current great names from other
leading medical institutions. This practice underscores symboli-
cally Pacific's great past, its current status, and its hopes for the
future. Its reputation for excellence attracts the top talent to both
Pacific's medical school and residency programs. By and large,
these recruits are considering careers in academic medicine; they
often have strong and well-defined research interests.

At one time, the splendor of Pacific's medical reputation was
matched by its physical setting in what was once the "gilded"
section of a large urban area. Most of the middle-class inhabi-
tants of the neighborhood have long since moved away and their
elegant mansions have been either leveled or subdivided into
many small apartments. The area that surrounds Pacific is
mostly lower-class black. This population generally uses the
emergency room at Pacific as its primary mode of obtaining
medical care. As a result, the surgical staff of Pacific sees many
patients who are in extreme pain and/or who are the victims of
traumas such as gunshot wounds, beatings, and stabbings. As a
consequence, a good number of the surgical patients at Pacific

meet their surgeons under conditions that are considerably less orderly than those for typical middle-class patients who are often referred after some diagnostic tests by their private physicians. As we shall see later, the nature of a patient's first meeting with the surgeon is often invoked to explain failure and/or error; however, for reasons I shall specify, such accounts are never accepted as legitimate excuses in themselves.

If the splendor of Pacific's neighborhood has faded, that of the hospital itself has not. Its central shell remains a magnificent Gothic structure with elaborate stonework, turrets, and gargoyles. Attached to the original building are several new wings of concrete and glass. The original square floor plan of the main building has with these additions become a bewildering maze of passageways, tunnels, and crosswalks linking old and new. The emergency room, the operating rooms, the surgical intensive care units, X ray, and the patient wards are all located on different floors in different parts of the hospital. Because of this, simply carrying out tasks in some logical order is often no mean feat.

Pacific is now approximately a 450-bed structure. Of those beds, 200 are allocated by the Admitting Office to general medicine and 193 to surgery. The remainder is for inpatient psychiatric services. Of the 193 beds allocated to the surgical services, approximately 120 are reserved for the surgical subspecialties such as neurosurgery, orthopedics, ENT (Ear, Nose, and Throat), plastics, cardiac and thoracic, and vascular. This leaves 75 beds or so for all four general surgery services which are the subject of this report. At Pacific, the general surgery services perform operations ranging in complexity from removal of hemorrhoids to esophagojejunostomies [an operation which binds the esophagus to the upper intestinal tract]. The general surgery services train housestaff to manage what are considered "normal, typical," surgical problems, and at the same time the services perform procedures which would not normally be undertaken elsewhere because of a patient's compromised condition, the lack of available support technology, or the presumptive lower level of competence and confidence of surgeons in other less elite institutions. The general surgery services have two classes of patients:

those referred from colleagues at Pacific or elsewhere because of the unusually complex nature of their problems, and those who entered through the emergency room. I did not observe that the two different types of patients received differential types of care. Attending surgeons in charge of services stress that they need an appropriate mix of both patients with complex and routine problems so that they can keep themselves challenged and at the same time give their housestaff adequate experience.

During the time of my observations, each of the four general surgery services performed an average of 24.5 major operations and 10.2 minor operations per week. The weekly mortality and morbidity rate, that is, the rate of death and complications, was 5.1. Our task here is not to evaluate whether this rate is high or low, but rather to explain what this rate means to two groups of participants, attending surgeons and surgical housestaff. In fact, one of our first tasks is to see what relationship, if any, exists between the morbidity and mortality rate—or the official rate of error—and the surgeon's construction of what an error is and what its seriousness is. A major focus of this inquiry, then, is the social processes invoked to construct these rates and the meaning these rates have for actors in this environment. In this context, it is interesting to note that each week the Department of Surgery at Pacific Hospital posts a list of deaths and complications by service, thereby distributing knowledge of misadventure very freely within its ranks.

I made observations on two different surgical services: first the Able and then the Baker (names and identifying characteristics have been altered). These two different services were chosen by the logic of the constant comparative method (Glaser and Strauss 1967). The general surgical services at Pacific Hospital varied in their approach to surgical work along a continuum, the poles of which were low clinical-high research orientation and high clinical-low research orientation. Able represented the high research end of the continuum, Baker the high clinical. The formal division of labor on each service was identical. At the top of the hierarchy were attending physicians, all of whom were full-time faculty of Pacific Medical College whose practices were limited to the patients on their service. At Pacific all patients were considered the private patients of the attendings whose service they were on: there were no surgical patients who were considered the housestaff's responsibility alone. In a strict legal sense, the attending surgeon was responsible for what happened to patients under his care. It was the attending who decided when to operate and what operation to perform. The attending surgeon was clearly the superordinate on the service. He was the final authority in any disagreements with housestaff; only the attending could give orders binding on every member of the service. Both the Able and the Baker Service had two attendings, each of whom had the final say for his patients. Attendings on a service might disagree with each other about patient care procedures, but each recognized the right of the other to treat his patients as he saw fit and proper.

On each service beneath the two attendings was a chief or senior resident. This resident was responsible for the day-to-day management of patients. He saw to it that the treatment plans of the attending for patients were carried out. The smooth running of the service—making sure that diagnostic tests occur on schedule, that patients do not run into any unexpected troubles, and that all work is done properly—is the chief or senior resident's responsibility. Essentially, he functioned as an attending in the attending's absence; his major task was to anticipate and treat problems before they occurred and to keep the attending informed of these actions. Beneath this level of authority are second- and third-year residents whose precise responsibilities are difficult to state. They must make sure the orders of the chief or senior resident are carried out. They lack responsibility for the entire service but have great responsibility for individual patients. Keeping medications straight, staying up to date on chart work, making certain the patient follows his postoperative regimen (usually walking and expanding the lungs to prevent pneumonia), and maintaining smooth working relations with nurses all seem to be part of this resident's responsibility.

At the bottom of the hierarchy are, in descending order, an intern, a senior medical student, and two or three junior medical students. To use a military analogy, these are the noncommissioned officers of the surgical world. The intern organizes the students so that the routine but necessary work (scut) of clinical care is done. Unlike the students, the intern can write medication orders and admit patients to the hospital. However, his authority in the hierarchical world of surgery is limited. Surgical interns often express resentment at how little they are allowed to take charge of. Senior medical students who may be contemplating surgical careers receive additional undergraduate exposure to surgery. For junior students, the surgery rotation is their first exposure to clinical surgical problems; for many who find surgery unappealing, it is also their last.

Each service varied at times in how it was staffed; there were variations in the number of individuals assigned to each service and in the ranks that were filled. On occasion, there were two second-year residents; at other times there was only one. On occasion, there were no senior students. The number of junior students varied between two and four. Variations in manpower were unrelated to patient load and were determined by the scheduling needs of graduate and undergraduate students. Whatever fluctuations existed in staffing, the formal tasks of both services were identical; preoperative and postoperative care, operating itself, evaluating referrals from other services, providing follow-up care to outpatients in the clinic, and supplying emergency room care and continuous coverage for patients of other services during "on-call" periods. The volume of work and the proportion of time devoted to each task varied, both among surgical services and within the same service for different time periods. Slack periods alternated with periods of frenzied activity. A brief description of the Able and Baker Services, excerpted from my field notes, follows.

The two attendings for Able Service, Dr. White and Dr. Peters, run the service from a distance. The two surgeons spend more time involved in their research activity than they do in direct clinical care of patients. Dr. White's main research interest is the problems surrounding organ transplantation. Maintaining the service allows him to control hospital beds for his kidney transplants. The activity of Able Service is geared to kidney transplants. Periods during which one or more transplants are being performed and/or managed are periods of peak activity; all members of the Able team are animated by a heightened sense of purpose. These periods contrast sharply with those when there are no transplants. Dr. Peters' major interest is research. Both Drs. White and Peters have excellent professional backgrounds and reputations, each having trained with a great name in American surgery. Attending rounds are made by Drs. White and Peters once a week on Saturday morning. They begin at nine in the morning and are over shortly after noon. Neither Dr. White nor Dr. Peters spends a great deal of time instructing residents in surgical techniques; only rarely do they run through a whole operation with subordinates. Chief residents are very active on Able Service; they have a great deal of decision-making power, they get to do a great deal of operating, and they are very much in charge. Residents and interns are not as a rule overly enthusiastic; they are critical of the range of cases that they see and of their actual operative experience. Students, especially those not heavily invested in a possible career in surgery, often relish being assigned to the Able Service since it has the reputation of being a "cakewalk." Dr. White feels that both he and Dr. Peters devote enough of their time and energy to clinical care:

> It all depends on what you mean. I know a lot of patients complain that they don't see us around; they think we're not concerned. What they don't understand is that just because we're not there doesn't mean that we don't know what's going on. I talk to X [current chief resident] every day and so does Peters. I have complete confidence in X. I've helped train him for the last five years. When the year started I really stood over his shoulder; but now I know that if he runs into anything that he can't handle, he'll call me. I live only fifteen minutes away. X can control the bleeding from the worst gunshot wound until I get here. Look, everybody expects Mehta to conduct the orchestra; but they don't expect him to play every instrument himself. Nobody criticizes Mehta when the oboe player hits a wrong note. Well, I lead the service. I don't do everything or watch everything and nobody expects me to. What I do expect is that my residents will keep me fully informed of everything that happens on my service.

The two attendings on the Baker Service, Drs. Arthur and Grant, spend more time involved in direct patient care than do the attendings on the Able Service. Most of Dr. Arthur's research publications are based on his clinical experiences. Dr. Grant does some laboratory work but his current research involves a large clinical series. The Baker Service has the reputation of dealing with the most difficult problems of the four general surgery services. Dr. Arthur specializes in diseases of the colon; Dr. Grant, the biliary tract. Dr. Arthur has a very powerful personality; many of his colleagues and residents think of him as an anachronism, a throwback to the time when surgeons were the prima donnas of the hospital. Dr. Arthur himself is aware of his reputation for theatricality but claims, "It is always well controlled. I use those tricks in very select cases in order to get a very specific response." He states that he learned this theatricality from the renowned surgeon for whom he was a resident. Dr. Grant, on the other hand, is more reserved. In most matters, Dr. Grant defers to Dr. Arthur. Attending rounds are made five days a week on the Baker Service by either Dr. Arthur, Dr. Grant, or both. The attendings use these rounds as their major teaching vehicle; in addition, Dr. Arthur holds a tumor conference once a week to discuss the management of cancer patients; and Dr. Grant meets with students on the service at least once a week to discuss general principles of surgery. Drs. Arthur and Grant are active in teaching surgical techniques to housestaff; they look over their subordinates' shoulders, running through the entire operation with them and giving lessons in basic anatomy to the others assembled in the operating room. Both Drs. Arthur and Grant do a lot of operating themselves. Occasionally, this is a source of tension for the service. Chief residents complain that they do not get enough cases. Residents and interns make the same complaint. By and large, however, housestaff like being assigned to the Baker Service. They state that they get an interesting mix of cases, that they are kept busy, and that both Drs. Arthur and Grant are superb teachers. Some housestaff express a distaste for the service because of Arthur's personality. The Baker Service is busier than the Able Service. It operates

more frequently than does Able; and for the period of observation, it had more inpatients and more requests for consultations.
Dr. Arthur explains his clinical emphasis as follows:

> Surgery is a body-contact sport, there is no question about it.
> You can't be a good armchair surgeon. If I want to know if
> my resident is doing a good job, I have to be in the operating
> room watching him. I can't tell what kind of a job a colleague
> has done from just looking at his patient. I may have suspi-
> cions but unless I was there and know what kind of situation
> he was presented with, I can't really say anything. There is no
> way of telling what kind of surgery was done without watching
> it. There is no way to teach surgery outside of the operating
> room that I know of—and I've been in this business a long
> time.

I made an initial assumption that was incorrect in a way that
proved serendipitous. I assumed that, both because of the different leadership styles of the Able and Baker attendings and
because of the different emphases of their services, I would have
a natural comparison of the ways errors were detected, coded,
and redressed in two different social groups, while holding the
task constant. However, no interactionally significant differences
emerged between the Able and the Baker Services in the handling
of errors. What was considered a serious breach on one service was
serious on the other. What was a trivial mistake on one service
was likewise trivial on the other. More strikingly, the phlegmatic
Dr. White and the theatric Dr. Arthur, given comparable
situations, tended to respond with the same degree of animation.
This alerted me to an underlying uniformity that informed the
surgical world view and I began to specify what the elements that
accounted for that uniformity were and how when taken together
they formed a unique *gestalt*. I began to feel that perhaps
Durkheim was more correct than he knew when he suggested that
each occupational group had its own unique morality.

During the period of field observation, I made the shared
problem that deaths and complications present the work group
and the shared and socially patterned ways that emerge for

meeting these difficulties the focus of my research. Since these problems do not arise on any scheduled basis, it was necessary for me to follow the schedule of a houseofficer in surgery in order to gather data. This involved following surgeons through their daily activities: I visited patients twice daily on rounds, drank coffee in the doctors' lounge during time-out periods, scrubbed in and assisted on operations when hands were short, stood over bodies as they were pronounced dead, and stayed on call at night and felt the rush of adrenalin that a life-threatening emergency brings.

I systematically varied the ways I interacted with the surgeons. On occasion, I actively questioned them about their actions; on others, I helped wheel the chart rack and medication cart on rounds, was available as a "gofer," and was as much as possible an extra pair of hands; on yet other occasions I observed as quietly as possible. I was by turns a more or less active participant in the scene. I could not correlate any set of roles I assumed with my informants' openness, that is, their willingness to share their thoughts and feelings on the unfolding social activity. The demands of medical work are so great and immediate and the field-worker is such a relatively unimportant figure in the clinical scheme of things that I felt my presence affected the phenomena I was interested in only in insignificant ways, if at all. Whatever the day-to-day or scene-to-scene shifts in the researcher persona, my overarching procedures did not vary. For two to three months, I would be totally immersed in fieldwork; I would go to the hospital six days a week and stay the course of the day. Notes were taken as soon after events as possible, routinely within twenty-four hours. Field notes attempted to record events in as narrative or straightforward fashion as possible. Then, after this intense immersion, I would leave the field for two weeks to a month and perform an "in situ" analysis of my field notes. I developed categories, interpretations, and hypotheses from the field notes and discovered where my data were weak and where my observations needed to be concentrated in the future. I then returned to the field for further observation. In this way I "saturated" my categories and "grounded" my theory (Glaser and Strauss 1967). I left the field only when I was convinced that my observations had reached the point of diminishing marginal utility.

Not all the problems I set for myself could be appropriately answered by data collected by participant observation alone. Among the questions I was interested in was the following: How consequential are negative sanctions to an individual's career path? To get at this question, I had to ask: How do superordinates, attending physicians, construct an evaluation of a houseofficer's competence from observations of the houseofficer's day-to-day task performance? I used two sources of data to supplement my field data: (1) I perused the written evaluations of housestaff by attending surgeons as contained in personnel files (to safeguard individual identities, to preserve confidentiality, all names and dates were removed from the documents before I received them), and (2) I attended the faculty meetings of the Department of Surgery at which the decision to retain or terminate junior housestaff in the training program is made. The process of this decision making has, to my knowledge, never been used in sociological studies of social control in the professions. This is an unfortunate omission since this is one of the few points in a professional career where controls exerted have a formal impact. These decisions serve to allocate medical manpower to different environmental niches in medical practice. The grounds on which these decisions are made reveal much about how effective we may expect the norms of medical culture to be in different environments and hence how effectively we may expect controls to operate.

Once fieldwork was completed, I interviewed those attendings and housestaff with whom I worked most closely. The interviews served two purposes. First, they served as a check on the validity of my data. Many of my interpretations were rephrased as questions for comment. In this way, I could match my assessments against those of actors in the scene; and I could fill in those spots where my observational material was thin. Second, the interviews allowed me to see my observations in a larger context. For example, housestaff were asked to compare their performance on different services. This provided me a fuller picture of their activity and their reaction to it than I could gather from my

field observations. Two different interview schedules were constructed: one for housestaff and one for attendings. These
schedules served as guides rather than formal instruments. All
interviews were kept as conversational as possible. Interviews
lasted between forty-five minutes and one and a half hours. For
attendings the focus of the interview was on how they decided if a
subordinate was good or bad and what they considered to be
unforgivable errors. Of housestaff, I asked what they thought
superordinate's performance expectations were, what they considered to be unforgivable errors, and what they considered the
major difficulties in becoming a surgeon.

I have collected data on the problem of deviance and social
control among general surgeons in a teaching hospital by a
number of methods: participant observation, perusal of staff
personnel folders, and interviews. I cataloged performance
from several different sources, in addition to my own observations. This triangulated approach to data gathering (see Webb et
al. 1966) gives me confidence in the validity of the inferences
which I have drawn. Often conclusions reached about performance from one data source are confirmed by another.

Theoretic Foundations

This is a field study that asks how surgeons recognize, define, punish, and/or neutralize failure. As a study of social control among
surgeons in an elite academic teaching hospital, this research
adds to our theoretical and empirical understanding of how the
quality of professional work is controlled. To answer these
questions about failure and error I utilize ethnographic methods.
So this study is also an ethnographic account of the ordinary and
extraordinary rites, rituals, and practices which comprise the
everyday life of surgeons. As ethnography this research provides,
I hope, a vivid, resonant description of behavior as it naturally
occurs. With ethnography properly done, ethnographic description has such a sense of verisimilitude, such a sense that "this
must be the way things happen," that the descriptive materials
provide a prima facie case for the validity of theoretic argument,

in this instance a discussion of the nature of social control in the medical profession. At times, unfortunately, the distinctive virtue of ethnography, its phenomenological richness, becomes a vice and one cannot see the theoretic forest for the too-richly described trees. As a result this ethnography, like so many others, runs the risk of being dismissed as "merely description" as if description itself were neither valuable nor necessary. In order to highlight as starkly as possible the way in which doing ethnography is always both a theoretic and a theoretically motivated activity, it is necessary to specify the theoretic and empirical questions that guided this research. After all, it was neither a love of surgeons nor of description that led to this study but rather my sense of what was deeply problematic about deviance, social control, and socialization in the sociology of the professions and the sociology of medicine.

When looking at the literature on deviance and social control in the professions, I have always been struck by the importance of the topic for various perspectives on the professions. Social control is the criterion variable that distinguishes one sociological perspective on the professions from another. Its analytic importance as a variable is matched by its empirical significance because of the policy implications that flow from how one conceptualizes professional behavior. If one follows Freidson, the doctor-patient relationship is an economic transaction in which the physician's primary motivation is to maintain a privileged and protected position for himself in the marketplace. If one follows Parsons, this relationship is one of fiduciary trust in which the physician's primary interest is to safeguard the health of the individual and collectivity. In large part, the policies one advocates at the macrolevel of state and profession are determined by the motivations one thinks operate on the microlevel of doctor and patient. In other words, whether or not the standard *caveat emptor* applies to the doctor-patient relationship is a question of profound sociological and empirical significance; any answer to this question is, of course, dependent on the degree to which the profession takes responsibility for its own social control.

However well or poorly the medical profession has managed

this responsibility, sociologists have analyzed the problem with neither rigor or subtlety. As Janowitz (1976) points out in another context, the term *social control* has had two quite distinct meanings in American sociology. On the one hand, the term is used to refer to an individual or group's capacity to regulate itself on its own initiative. On the other hand, it also refers to the coercive means at a community's disposal to discipline individuals. All of that is to say, social control may be internal or external. It is important to emphasize here that the internal controls are not merely individual or group intrapsychic processes—a family that settles its own disputes, or a work group that disciplines its own members are examples of groups ordered by internal social controls. Furthermore, social control may be formal (judicial process) or informal (an off-the-cuff rebuke). Combining these two dimensions we can derive four analytically distinct modalities of social control.

Informal-internal social controls are the everyday ways that members of a group remind each other of their responsibilities as part of their work routines. For example, as anyone who has had an impulse checked by an innocent question can attest, ordinary conversation exerts a greatly underrated and unappreciated force as a source of control.

All groups possess *formal-internal* means for periodically reviewing their performance. Such institutionalized review varies according to frequency, consequences, formality, and so on. Formal-internal social controls may be blunted by the need and/or desire to sustain pleasant working relations with colleagues. Nevertheless, formal accountability is a regular feature of group life. The case conference in psychiatry, the brown-bag lunch in sociology departments, staff meetings in a bureaucracy —all serve either implicitly or explicitly a social control function.

External controls are those where the individual or group that monitors, judges, and sanctions behavior is neither the individual nor a member of the group whose performance is under scrutiny. The principal who drops in on classrooms, the teacher who gives a surprise quiz, the mother-in-law who visits unannounced in the middle of the day are all using the tactics of *informal-external* control. Such controls are a privilege of rank, which is why school principals are able to employ this method more successfully than mothers-in-law. Random checks are seen by control agents as a particularly effective method of monitoring performance since the performance observed cannot be staged for the occasion. By the same token, those subject to them fear such spot checks since they leave so much to chance.

The official audit is the paradigm of *formal-external* control. Here, there is a regular, ongoing review of performance, standards of acceptable performance are set in advance on the basis of objective criteria, and negative sanctions are attached to failures to meet expectations. Such control mechanisms are highly efficient means for monitoring performance. There appears to be an inverse relationship between moral credibility and formal-external controls: parolees are subject to quite a few, judges virtually none.

In treating social control in the professions, sociologists have not kept even these rather rudimentary dimensions of the term distinct. There is an inability to distinguish internal from external controls and formal from informal ones. Discussing social control in medicine, sociologists have consistently written as if some part stood for the whole. Studies of socialization, deviance, and social control have concentrated on one aspect or another of the paradigm sketched above but they have not seen how the components of it are interrelated nor have they paid close attention to the link between the socialization of physicians and the system of social control.

It is in studies of the socialization of medical students and houseofficers that sociologists have most concentrated on the informal-internal aspects of the work environment. The work of Becker et al. (1961) detailed the processes by which groups of students act in concert to restrict their production as a reaction to what were felt to be the unrealistic and overly burdensome demands of faculty. The Kansas study concentrated rather exclusively on the allocation of student effort and ignored other problems for which students forge collective solutions, such as what is ethical behavior, what is acceptable practice, what makes a colleague trustworthy. Fox (1957a, 1963), in her studies of medical socialization, analyzed how medical students learned to manage their uncertainties and how they learned to strike a balance between detachment and concern. Like Becker, Fox concentrates on the informal-internal cues the student receives from the environment; and, like Becker, Fox neglects to connect this socialization to the area of deviance and social control, especially the individual's latter capacity to monitor, evaluate, and correct his/her own performance. Since internal controls are often learned through informal, if often systematic, ways, and since routines of a work group both establish and enforce the background expectancies against which action is viewed as proper or not, it is clear that a refined theory of social control needs to attend to these phenomena.

The formal-internal mechanisms of social control among physicians have been treated by both Goss (1961) and Freidson and Rhea (1972, 1975). They have observed that such reviews control bureaucratic conditions of work and not the work itself. Direct orders never seem to be given; negative sanctions are rarely, if ever, applied; and advice is offered haltingly, without any attempt to see if it is followed up. Social control mechanisms reinforced by negative sanctions seem not to exist. Such a system either protects the inept, as Goode (1967) suggests, and/or rests on strongly shared norms that presuppose self-corrective action. From the analyses provided we are not in a position to evaluate which of the above is the case, nor are we in a position to assess how these controls are related to those built into everyday activity.

Stelling and Bucher (1972) have described informal-external review. They describe an elaborate set of tactics by subordinates to resist encroachments on their autonomy and a correspondingly elaborate set of countermoves by superordinates to gather information on staff performance. Their discussion of interactional strategies—informative as it is—neglects phenomenological aspects of monitoring: Which acts lead to increased monitoring? What other more enduring negative sanctions go along with increased monitoring? How universal and uniform are the standards that different superordinates apply?

Finally, the absence of formal-external controls—regular audit of practitioner performance or regular recertification—has led sociologists to conclude that if juridical-type controls do not exist then no social controls exist at all. A recent spate of prescriptive treatises in the sociology of medicine (Barber et al. 1973; Crane 1975; Freidson 1975; Gray 1975) all make a similar argument: namely, since the profession itself does not have a well-articulated system of formal controls then regulatory responsibility must be removed from the profession or at least structurally formalized. Whatever the merits of such a strategy—and they are considerable—its rationale rests on the decidedly asociological proposition that the only effective social control is coercive or formal control. Totally dismissed is the notion that individual control or group pressure effectively constrains behavior. It seems to me possible to argue for a more formal system of controls while acknowledging the substantial amount of control that is built into the system through socialization, work routines, and normal relations with colleagues. It is precisely this that a professional dominance perspective fails to do.

There is already a great deal that we know about socialization, deviance, and social control in the medical profession. We know that much role learning takes place informally among peers and that this learning includes aspects of the role that can be evaded as well as those obligations which are sacrosanct. We know that internal regulation concerns more an individual's organization of his/her effort than the quality of that effort. We know that subordinates evade monitoring and superordinates know about and plan for this evasion. We know that colleagues are hesitant about confronting other colleagues with their misdeeds and even more hesitant about applying negative sanctions. We know that an institutionalized system of punishments is so rarely resorted to that for all practical purposes it can hardly be said to exist. We know that some physicians show great dedication, duty, and tirelessness as they pursue their tasks, while others merely go through the motions. We know that those who speak for the profession as a whole are aware that they have within their ranks the slothful, the mendacious, the untrustworthy, and the out-

and-out corrupt; yet corporate remedies for these professional problems are slow to emerge.

There is no debating that the number of coercive or external controls that the medical profession imposes on its members is few. Likewise the number of formal controls that operate is few. Does this mean that controls are entirely absent? If so, how are young physicians socialized to explain away their failures? If not, what are the informal-internal controls? How effective are they? What are their limitations? And how do they articulate with other modalities of control? When the medical profession claims that it controls itself, what does it mean? Is it claiming that its individual members each regulate him/herself so well that any additional controls are unnecessary, or is it claiming that what corporate controls exist are adequate for the task? If the first is the case, how is this remarkable feat achieved; if the second is the case, how do we know? This ethnography explores socialization and social control from the point of view of the surgeon in the teaching hospital. It is an analytical rather than a total ethnography. By this I mean that it is not an attempt to order as fully as possible all dimensions of the surgeon's experience. It is instead a very select crosscut of the surgeon's world in order to answer a very specific empirical question with important theoretical implications, the empirical question being how is social control achieved in this particular environment? I began by taking mortality and morbidity as an indicator of situations in which controls might be appropriate and tried to see from this starting point what physicians regard as an error and what criterion they use to construct error as an objectively given real event, rather than as the arbitrary outcome of any number of independent judgments in an indeterminate sequence of judgments. I am interested in how the physician as a practical theorist establishes "this is what the objects in my world are and this is how they behave," and I am interested in the play of claim and counterclaim by participants in interaction to establish that this is real, this is what happened, this is the way it happened, this is why it happened.

Strange as it seems, what an error is has not been problematic in previous studies of social control in medicine. Previous studies have assumed that what counts as an error is a relatively straightforward matter. This is to say that the studies apply, or imply physicians can and should apply, a standard criterion in identifying error. Error, the object of and cause for social control, belongs to a class of events with such readily identifiable characteristics that on any occasion its recognition is deemed unproblematic. An event possesses the requisite characteristics and fits the class or it does not. Moreover, these attributes are specified in advance of the fact and not determined in a retrospective or ex post facto fashion. In the literature it is taken for granted that what counts as an error is easily recognized and agreed on by all concerned. What is problematic is whether such events will be punished or go undisciplined. Now, this categorical view of error displays both a misapprehension of the nature of medical decision making and of the interactional dynamics which surround social control in a profession.

Medical decision making is a probabilistic enterprise. Presented with a patient with a set of symptoms, the physician makes a diagnosis and decides on an intervention. Only rarely is it the case in which the physician can say "this patient has x and we must do y." Even when it is certain that a patient has x, this does not dictate what should be done since the treatment of choice will vary according to the severity of x, the patient's age, the physician's skill, and the technology available at any given hospital. Moreover, there are some disorders for which there is significant disagreement among equally learned colleagues over what the treatment of choice should be. Finally it is not always clear that a patient has x since there are any number of disorders with similar symptoms. Whatever may be the nature and depth of his uncertainty, the physician is usually forced by the patient's condition to act before that uncertainty is resolved. In this situation, the physician's action is dictated by what he knows at the time. I am not denying that there are diagnostic errors made during the initial contact of physician and patient and that some of these are sustained until the patient's death. What I am saying is that not all diagnoses and treatments that later experience proves wrong are mistakes; some are actions that any reasonable physician would have made under the circumstances. It is plainly not possible to understand how the social controls in the medical profession operate unless one understands how physicians draw the line between what was a reasonable treatment option that subsequent events proved wrong and a course of action that was indefensible given the facts at hand, an error.

Because we as medical sociologists have not understood the difference between these two types of events, because we have given error an unequivocal ontological status, we have missed a step in analyzing the negotiated order of social control. The characteristic slowness of, the hesitation surrounding, and the lenience of professional control in medicine has been well documented; but how physicians view such practices and why they allow them has not. What counts as an error—that set of background understandings, norms, and values that are invoked to categorize clinical events as blameworthy error or blameless misfortune—has not been explored. We have been quite glib in describing how errors are treated, but we have neglected to explain what errors are. The sociologist's understanding of error diverges in a fundamental way from the physician's. For the physician, error is what W. J. Gallie (Lukes 1977) calls an "essentially contested" concept. By this term, Gallie means to convey the inevitable indeterminateness of certain socially constructed categories, such as beautiful or merciful. There are grounds for debating the appropriateness of these concepts on each and every occasion of their use. For the physician, error is just such an essentially contested concept. In this report, I first ask how error is defined, by whom, and under what circumstances; and then I ask how it is managed. Because of my extensive and intensive field experience, I am able to do this from the point of view of others—the surgeon who has made an error, the surgeon who has discovered one made by a colleague, and the surgeon who is responsible for seeing that such a breach is both corrected and not repeated. I do not take the point of view of the patient since the occurrence of error is usually concealed from him and since he does not enter the interactions which surround social control. However lamentable the fact, the patient is an exogenous variable falling outside the system of social control.

While starting with the question of what is error rather than how it is managed does not appear a momentous matter, it promises to advance our understanding of the professions, both as occupations with the special privileges and burdens of rank, as collectivities with rituals for celebration and for mourning, and as fraternities with means to close ranks for self-protection and preservation. By asking what an error for a surgeon is in particular and for a physician in general, I avoid prejudging the adequacy of the modes of social control, but concentrate instead on how this activity is accomplished. Moreover, raising the question in this fashion allows me to explore some recurrent issues on the nature of professions in our society. First, there is a general consensus among sociologists that professions are distinct from other occupational groups by their claims of both a body of theoretic knowledge on which practice rests and a special code of conduct which governs relations among colleagues, clients, and the general public. It follows then that there are two possible sources of deviance. On the one hand, there is the body of theoretic knowledge. Mistakes are made in either judgment or the application of techniques. On the other hand, there is the code of conduct on which professional practice rests. Mistakes are made in the interpretation of norms, that is, the moral standards of the community. Are mistakes, whatever their source, treated the same or is one type of mistake treated more seriously than the other? Do those two types of events occur with equal frequency?

Second, although many sociologists have indicated in a very general way the range of responses to error among physicians, they have failed to link performances to sanctions—that is, they have engaged the issue of social control only after physicians have made the diagnosis of colleague error. I ask by what criteria do surgeons make this diagnosis and what treatments do they view as appropriate given such a diagnosis. My goal is to make clear the fit between the type of error and the type of response it provokes in a community of professionals.

Third, we do not know what types of "recovery work" physicians are forced to do to make failure excusable nor do we know what kinds of failure are considered unforgivable. Given the diffuse uncertainty that surrounds medical diagnosis and decision making, errors attributable to the body of theoretic knowledge may be more easily neutralized than those attributable to the code of conduct since presumably there is much less uncertainty here. Even so, it may be the case that each type of error has its own specific mode of recovery work unique to it. Certainly there are mistakes that physicians make from which patients never recover. Are there mistakes which physicians make from which they themselves cannot recover, which are fatal to their careers and their standing in their colleague community? What are these?

Fourth, we do not understand the effects of available punishments and controls on career paths. Sociologists have long been interested in career paths; in high-status, highly competitive fields such as medicine and surgery, we often make the assumption that one earns one's position. Should we not also entertain the idea that some career niches are a form of exile and punishment, whatever the material rewards, and that some physicians inhabit these niches as a result of professional misdeeds? I explore how social controls sort physicians into different work and career spaces. I examine how consequential the everyday evaluation of performance is for the physician's career. Do negative sanctions have very short-lived effects or do their effects live on and affect a physician's entire career?

Fifth, we do not know how recruits to a profession learn what the standards of performance are, learn the difference between forgivable and unforgivable failure, and learn for themselves how to interpret professional license and mandate. By observing the social control of error among surgical housestaff I can explicate a neglected dimension of medical socialization; namely, how a physician forms his sense of what is professionally right and wrong. During training one learns how to discriminate humanely avoidable from absolutely inevitable failure; how in the case of avoidable failure to distinguish between innocent and blameworthy mistakes; and how, in the case of blameworthy mistakes, to do penance for misdeeds. This is to say, that through socialization, a professional superego develops, models of acceptable behavior are formed, and models of atoning for unacceptable behavior are learned. We assume that these models exert a continuing influence throughout an individual's career—their strength being contingent on their reinforcement in the workplace. However, we know little of their continuing influence because we know so little about the formation of the norms of clinical practice.

In short, our lack of understanding of how physicians detect, categorize, and punish error is fatal to our understanding of social control in the medical profession. Because of this, we do not know how to interpret a profession's claim to be self-regulating. We have no idea of the interplay of event, claim, and counterclaim from which professional deviance and social control is constructed. In this report, I shall look at the patterns of behavior that determine whether an event is labeled an error or not; examine the factors that determine the gravity of an error, independent of its effect on a patient; analyze how individual actors understand the rules for labeling error; and see how these rules help form a hierarchical, but very limited authority system which has very concrete implications for the quality of care we all receive.

Why Surgeons?

A fair question at this point is, Why study one group of surgeons at one elite teaching hospital in order to determine how error is detected, categorized, and punished among physicians? Has sociology as a discipline not developed techniques that lead to generalizations that are valid for a larger population and that lend themselves to easier replication? To argue for some approach to this problem other than an ethnographic one misses much of what I have had to say thus far about the nature of medical decision making and errors. My choice of method, site, and subject was guided first and foremost by theoretic concerns. I have argued that error is an "essentially contested" concept. By this I mean that the grounds for fixing the label "error" to any action are always arguable. In two similar cases with identical outcomes one person may be considered guilty of an error while the other is blameless. Our task in this report is to account for this difference. We need to see under what circumstances, by what criteria, with what consequences, for which audiences an act is or is not considered an error. There is quite simply no other way to do this other than by observing physicians as they account for cases where outcomes fall short of expectations. In this way alone can we determine on what grounds the label "error" is contested and what grounds are essential to establish the label.

Even so, the logic that dictates a field study, that is, the vague, relative, and emergent qualities of the category "error," does not compel us to look at surgeons. We could just as well observe psychiatrists (a favorite pursuit of sociologists) or cardiologists or neurologists or dermatologists. We could look at two or three specialties and compare the way errors are treated within them. However, there are qualities peculiar to the practice of surgery that make surgeons the most appropriate object of our study. In fact, these same qualities allow surgeons to be singled out by critics of health care as it is currently organized as prime abusers of the public trust. Impressive statistics on unnecessary surgery, highly publicized malpractice settlements, sensational media accounts of criminal incompetence and neglect have all combined to make the surgeon a dramatic symbol of what is wrong with the profession of medicine. There is some poetic justice in this. After all, the surgeon who performs under a spotlight in an operating theater was for years the prima donna in the hospital and the object of public adulation. Parsons (1951) has even suggested that surgeons as instrumentally active, pragmatically oriented individuals who take decisive action to save human life display value patterns and behaviors that are emblematic of the "hero" in American society. Worthy of note in this respect are the many popular culture presentations of physicians that feature surgeons such as Ben Casey, Joe Gannon, or the M.A.S.H. medics. We are all familiar with the de rigeur nature of the decisive operation in hospital drama. The features of surgery that make surgeons "heroes" from one point of view at one point in time and that make them symbols of corruption, mendacity, and greed from another point of view at another time are the very features that make surgeons so well suited to serve as subjects of this report. These features are the precise and definitive nature of surgical intervention—its visibility, the expectation of success that surrounds this intervention, and the relatively short time frame in which outcomes are known. All of these make surgeons more accountable than their colleagues in other specialties.

Surgical interventions are very precise and definitive. The surgeon cuts into the body and removes or rearranges various body parts in order to cure or palliate disease. For patients, surgery is intrusive and radical therapy. The specific nature of surgical treatment links the action of the physician and the response of the patient more intimately than in other areas of medicine. In many branches of internal medicine the physician's interventions are relatively nonspecific. This fact allows internists to attribute failure to the inevitable pathophysiology of the disease process rather than to the nature of treatment itself. In psychotherapy, where goals are often diffuse and treatment is neither precise nor definitive, Light (1972) has demonstrated that in cases of failure the actions of therapist and the response of the patient are not seen as linked. Light reports that the normative belief that the patient alone is responsible for his actions and his life is routinely invoked following suicide, when the imputation of therapist error is strongest. Precise, definitive interventions with very specific expectations make failure to achieve objectives a more salient issue than in areas where interventions are nonspecific and expectations diffuse. Of all physicians, the surgeon's interventions are most visible and his therapeutic expectations are most specific. These features intimately link the surgeon's action to the patient's condition.

So clearly are the surgeon's actions connected to the patient's condition that the only warrant for surgery—the only acceptable reason to subject a patient to the risk and trauma of surgery—is the expectation that the operation will cure or palliate the patient's condition. The expectation of success is the background understanding which legitimates surgical action. Such an expectation does not govern action to the same degree in other specialties. To understand this point, let us compare two examples. If a surgeon operates on an eighty-three-year-old patient with gallbladder problems and the patient dies, then the surgeon cannot very well make the claim that the patient died of old age. He must first explain how and why the patient received a scar on his abdomen. Now, an internist medically managing the same gallbladder problem with the same result can legitimately claim that the patient died of old age. Deaths and complications present different questions to different specialists. When the patient of an internist dies, the natural question his colleagues ask is, "What happened?" When the patient of a surgeon dies his colleagues ask, "What did you do?" By the nature of his craft and his beliefs about it, the surgeon is more accountable than other physicians and he also has much more to account for. Of course, this is not all to say that every time a surgical patient dies the surgeon is at fault, only that it is much harder for him to claim that he had no hand in it than it is for other colleagues.

The expectation of success which is the only warrant for surgery compels the surgeon to be more sensitive than his colleague to the implicit indictment of his skill and/or judgment signified by therapeutic failure. But to say that there is an expectation of success is to recognize the possibility of failure. In a very real way every time a surgeon operates, he is making book on himself. Besides the enormous amount of theoretic and technical expertise that is his cognitive capital, the surgeon carries in his head an odds-book for each procedure he performs; he knows the mortality and morbidity attached to each procedure; and he is able to revise these odds up or down on the basis of each patient's age and physical condition. The risk taking implicit in surgical action makes surgical failure a double-edged sword: one may avoid charges of technical incompetence only to be accused of reckless judgment. Because of the nature of the surgeon's risk taking on the patient's behalf, a comprehensive look at surgeons lays bare many social and ethical dilemmas which modern medicine faces. Among these are How is the

Hippocratic injunction, "First, do no harm" to be interpreted? What is acceptable risk? How are scarce healing resources allocated? What constitutes informed consent? What is the trade-off between technical virtuosity and compassionate healing?

Because of the visibility of their actions and the expectations that surround them, each death and complication raises the question of error and responsibility for surgeons in a very direct way. By observing the shared and socially patterned ways that surgeons treat deaths and complications, we shall see how surgeons discover and label failure, how they attempt to avoid the implicit indictment of their skills attendant upon failure, and how they punish whoever are deemed culpable parties. However, I am not just observing any surgeons, but surgeons in an elite, academic enviroment. It is reasonable to ask, How is this practice setting distinct from more modal ones? First, increased account-ability is generic to surgery, but it is possible that mechanisms for actually achieving this accountability are not equally present in all practice settings. I assume—and my informants report—that both formal and informal mechanisms for achieving account-ability are more available in elite than in nonelite settings. To be elite means to assume a stance of "first among equals." In elite settings the practice of surgery focuses on difficult surgical cases that represent what is presumptively "the cutting edge" of the field; the major concern is for the elegance of surgery—its artful dimensions—uncontaminated by such mundane matters as fees and their collection, social exchanges to generate referrals, and so on. Where preeminenece is unquestioned, there may be a greater willingness to explore the reasons for failure. This is all the more so in an academic environment which encourages technical talk about a case in a theoretic manner so that unfortunate results may be detached from those that caused them.

There is a second reason for assuming that mechanisms of social control are more prevalent in our setting. Apart from the consequences of its elite reputation, Pacific is an academic institution. Ranks of superordinates and subordinates are quite distinct; the hierarchy is extremely visible and is known to all. Since a part of any socialization process is both positive and negative reinforcement, we would expect the informal-internal processes of control to occur more commonly in teaching institutions. We would expect this quite apart from the fact that superordinates can and do limit subordinates more easily than they do colleagues. So our site, we assume, differs from more modal settings in that at the very least the very processes that we were most interested in would be more present than in other settings. I assume that the general patterns I found hold in all settings. For example, I found that what I call technical errors are always subordinated to what I call normative errors. I assume that this is true for all settings. What I do not know is how universal versus how situated professional norms are; so as a consequence, I cannot describe whether the norms of Pacific's surgeons are shared only by other members of the academic elite or by all surgeons. This is certainly an important issue, but it does not alter the general argument that I make about the relation of individual to corporate controls in the profession nor does it alter the arguments I make about how the legitimacy of quasi-normative or idiosyncratic standards undermine the control process. My site selection limits the universe to which I can generalize, but at the same time it provides a setting in which controls are both salient and displayed in their most primitive form. It allows us to see most clearly what surgeons consider an error, why they use this definition, and how they enforce it.

Conclusion and Overview

I have argued that discussions of social control in medicine and the professions are flawed because they take what an error is for granted. Such studies ignore the phenomenological nature of error as a category of social life and the probabilistic nature of medical decision making. I have attempted to remedy this defect through a field study of surgeons at Pacific Hospital, an elite urban institution. I spent my time on two different services; first, the Able—a high research–low clinical orientation unit; and then, the Baker—a high clinical–low research orientation unit. During my fieldwork, I made failure in the everyday life of the physician and the shared and socially patterned ways that emerge for dealing with it my focal concern. I explain how failure is recognized, managed, controlled, and denied. Since by virtue of their task structure and norms of accountability failure is such a salient question for surgeons, I made them the subjects of my inquiry.

In the next chapter, I will explore the various interpretations of failure that surgeons routinely employ. Four definitions categorize failure—technical error, judgmental error, normative error, and quasi-normative error. Normative and quasi-normative errors alone challenge a surgeon's claim of competence. Chapter 2 shows how these definitions of failure are negotiated and how these labels for failure are related to the division of labor. We are concerned here with the articulations of the division of labor and responsibility.

I turn, in chapter 3, to the various everyday methods superordinates employ to keep error at a minimum. I shall show how these control tactics involve encroaching on the autonomy of subordinates; and I shall describe how subordinates resent and resist this encroachment. In so doing, I shall explore the tension between the two competing systems of legitimation in the medical world: rule by clinical experience and rule from scientific evidence. Second, I examine the questioning process that superordinates use to assign errors to one category or another. Third, I shall analyze the "horror story" as a key element in the oral culture of the medical world and show how it functions as a social control mechanism.

Chapter 4 explores formal peer review in surgery. In this chapter, I show how surgeons account for the "normal troubles" of their craft. I develop a paradigm that allows us to typify these normal troubles and to show the tactics of interpretation surgeons use as a routine part of the "recovery work" for failure. I then analyze a peculiar ritual which occurs in formal peer review sessions: "putting on the hair shirt." Here, superordinates admit error and humble themselves before an audience of colleagues and subordinates. I shall explain the nature of these ritualized admissions of fallibility.

In chapter 5, I explore the impact of failure on a subordinate's career path. I shall show what breaches the surgical profession considers tolerable, and what breaches are unforgivable. I shall explore how the day-to-day performance of subordinates is evaluated and how the judgment "this is a promising surgeon" is constructed. In this analysis we can see the operation of license and mandate collapsed into a single act: the promotion and dismissal of recruits.

Chapter 6 concludes the study by showing how professional self-control operates. I show how professional deviance is identified. I demonstrate how controls operate. I assess one consequence of this definition of the situation: the hypertrophy of individual controls and the atrophy of corporate control. I also present a methodological appendix which describes how I collected and coded my data and how I made myself a part of the surgeon's routine environment.

two

Error, Rank, and Responsibility

When deaths and complications disturb the surgical expectation of success, those involved are compelled to find good reasons to account for failure.[1] A grammar of motives is manipulated to find an acceptable answer to the question, What went wrong?[2] Moreover, deaths and complications are only one way in which surgical action is disrupted. Nurses and housestaff quarrel; diagnostic procedures do not occur as scheduled; patients fail to follow surgical regimens; and worried families disturb what are, for the physician, the most prosaic of procedures with questions, requests for more information, and demands for reassurance. All of these activities—in addition to the failure of surgical intervention itself —lead attending surgeons to question a houseofficer's competence. None of these events is a failure in and of itself, but all such events carry failure's frightening imputations. These events are occasions for negotiating whether a failure did in fact occur, whether that failure is a result of individual error, and whether or not that error is excusable.

The failure to sustain orderly surgical activity[3] varies in intensity as a threat to a subordinate's competence, depending on how rudely expectations are breached, how frequently an individual breaches expectations, and how easily, if at all, the action may be reversed. This chapter explores the meanings that are negotiated in the wake of breached expectations, relates these meanings to the division of labor, and explores how these meanings are fateful for those involved. The explanation of failure has far-reaching ramifications since it morally typifies the person who is considered responsible. My concern here is with only the informal working understandings of superiors and subordinates that sustain continued action in the face of failure. Later I will discuss formal negotiations, as they occur in peer review, and formal evaluations of performance, as they occur among attending surgeons when tracking housestaff into different career paths.

A surgeon's attempts to explain preventable failure may be divided into four categories: (1) technical error, (2) judgmental error, (3) normative error, and (4) quasi-normative error. Although other interpretations of failure exist, only these four categories deal directly with the issue of physician competence and the social control of performance. Other labels are an attempt to locate responsibility in an area outside the surgeon's control, and are thus often of questionable legitimacy because of the highly developed ethic of individual responsibility among surgeons.

Technical Errors

When a surgeon makes a technical error, he is performing his role conscientiously but his skills fall short of what the task requires. Technical errors are expected to happen to everyone, but rarely. They are expected to happen to everyone because surgeons understand that theirs is at best an imperfectly applied science. At times, interventions fail because techniques have been less than perfectly performed. Certain failures of technique are expected as a routine and calculable part of the work environment: they are built into training. Knots tied by the unpracticed may leave dead space for infection or may split; probes and scopes in the hands of the inexperienced may explore more of the body than desired:

> There are always complications from unfamiliar techniques. A resident may get a pneumothorax [air or gas introduced into the pleural cavity] when he taps a chest, or he may get a hematoma [a large bruise] after a procedure. If these things didn't happen to him, he wouldn't need us; he'd already be a professor of surgery. These things still happen to me but not nearly so often. They are the reason we have a training program, so housestaff can learn to do procedures without incident (Attending).[4]

Further, attending surgeons claim that they can forgive even the most serious lapses in technique, the grossest of mistakes:

Look, suppose when a resident opens the abdomen he nicks the aorta—now that's dumb, stupid, anything you want to call absolute incompetence; I mean, the only way to do that is to really dig in with the knife. It's plain dumb, but it's not unforgivable. It's a mistake and everybody makes mistakes one way or another. Our job is to minimize these mistakes and give people the kind of training that makes them rare (Attending).

Certain failures are then interpreted as technical in nature. They are seen by attendings as an occasion for passing on to apprentice surgeons the "tricks of the trade." Such failures highlight a training definition of the situation. In cases of technical error, the role-relation of attending and houseofficer is that of teacher and student.

For an error to be defined as technical, two conditions must be met. First the error has to be speedily noticed, reported, and treated. Such a chain of events serves as a signal of the subordinate's good intentions at the same time that it allows treatment of the problem before it becomes unmanageable. The same objective condition reported immediately on one occasion and later on another will meet with a different response from attendings. Given the inevitability of problems, their speedy report underscores a houseofficer's conscientiousness and his concern for the patient; it pays tribute to the norms of clinical responsibility at the same time that events themselves mock these norms. As we shall see, a slow discovery of a technical error leads attendings to suspect that more than a technical failure was involved; they begin to think a moral lapse may have been involved as well. Moreover, quick reporting of error maximizes the possibility of routine remedies and thus minimizes for all the cost of failure.

We left Julio Jimenez's room after rounds. Mark, the chief resident, shook his head and spoke: "I had bad dreams about Julio all night. He's got this horrible infection going on in his belly; and I can't figure out what's causing it. This infection is clearly the result of some technical error. It could have been caused by any of a multitude of factors, really. But it's a technical error, no doubt about it. Fortunately, for us and for

him, Carl [the intern] noticed it right away or else he'd be
awfully sick and we'd have a real mess on our hands"
(Able Service).

It is nevertheless important to remember that the costs of
technical failure never shrink to zero, and it is the patient who
always pays. The patient pays financially in increased hospital
costs and pays personally in the discomfort of a complication. For
subordinates, quick report of failure is one of the primary means
of establishing that the error is not representative of its maker,
that it signals only a momentary lapse, and that it occurred
merely because of its maker's inexperience.

A second condition must be met for failure to be defined as
technical; mistakes must not be frequently made by the same
person. When an individual makes mistakes frequently, he cannot legitimately claim that a momentary lapse occurred. Moreover, attendings would not accept such a claim because frequent
failure makes them doubt not only a subordinate's efforts but also
his intentions:

> When a person makes the same mistake over again, you know
> you're not getting through. For example, if a person comes
> into the operating room and he's tying knots improperly, then
> you tell him, "You practice tying knots on your bedpost and
> not my patient." And if the next time you're in the operating
> room he's doing the same thing, you can see that he's not
> making progress. And if he's not applying himself in one
> area, he's probably not applying himself in others (Attending).

In fact, when an error occurs, attendings ask themselves how
often this housestaff member has been involved in this sort of
thing:

> When you see residents make a mistake, you ask yourself:
> "Are they repeating the same mistake?" It's a matter of
> memory. To be frank, it's holding a grudge. I'm sure you've
> heard us say: "Forgive and remember." When you see some-
> thing, you ask yourself: "Has that happened before? Is it a
> pattern?" (Attending).

For their part, housestaff are worried not so much about making a mistake as failing to learn from those mistakes that they do make. They report, almost universally, the same feelings: at the beginning of their training they are terribly afraid that they will make errors that will have disastrous consequences for patients. Then they learn that they and all those around them make mistakes and that generally the consequences of such mistakes can be managed. Finally, they fear repeating the same mistakes and not learning from their experience. However, all report that their errors are etched indelibly in their memory:

> Of course I worry about making a mistake and it really being disastrous for a patient. But really the crime is not making a mistake; everybody is going to make mistakes. The crime is not learning from your errors. What is really inexcusable is making the same mistake twice. For example, once I can remember sending home a young girl who came into the emergency room at four in the morning and who had abdominal pains and couldn't urinate. I was lucky somebody read over what I had done the next day and said: "Good God, get her back right away—she has appendicitis." So they brought her back and operated that afternoon and she did have appendicitis. That was a case of me not knowing enough and making the wrong decision, but nothing like that will happen again. I learned from it (Intern).

> Mistakes bother you less and less as you go on. I was really sensitive when I started. Fear of doing something wrong and being yelled at was a real motivating factor for me at first. I combatted the fear by working hard and paying a lot of attention to detail. During training you find out mistakes are not such a bad thing and that everybody makes them. But my first year I was extremely afraid. I became less afraid as I went along, but I also made fewer mistakes because I had more experience (Chief Resident).

This knowledge—that a mistake once made should never be made again—is a commonsense understanding that allows both housestaff and attendings to face the unpleasant fact that, because they carried out a task less than competently, another individual was caused to suffer. Technical errors and their lessons are even transformed on occasion into positive experiences. Benefits of the error are believed to outweigh the costs. One individual suffers, but legions of patients yet unseen have the lesson gleaned from this error passed on to them. Moreover, attendings need a certain number of errors in order to teach housestaff how to avoid common problems or how to meet them when they arise. Housestaff need exposure to a wide range of problems so that when training is completed, they are prepared to meet any of the contingencies which disrupt surgical action.

Be that as it may, neither attendings nor housestaff are sanguine in the face of technical error; and every effort is made to keep the number of technical errors small. While the acceptance of technical error is easy as a long-run and abstract proposition, concrete instances are most unwelcome. Work is organized on a surgical service in order to suppress the absolute number of technical errors. Two factors are most noteworthy. First, there is the technical division of labor which is arranged so that subordinates do not advance to complex tasks until they have demonstrated their competence at simpler ones. Before doing nonoperative procedures on their own for the first time, housestaff are shown how by more experienced service members and they are routinely monitored the first time they perform a task. Operations are performed by housestaff under the watchful eyes of attendings or more experienced residents who give advice during the procedure. So much is this supervision expected that when it does not occur, subordinates feel abandoned by superordinates:

> Paul, a second-year resident, was to perform his first colostomy [opening and externalizing a segment of the colon] on Mr. Herman, a patient with cancer of the rectum. Dr. Peters, Mr. Herman's attending, entered the room before the procedure began and asked Paul if he had ever done one of these before. Paul said he hadn't. Peters told him it would be no problem, that they would whip right through it. Peters then took a marking pencil and drew a line on Herman's abdomen indicating how he'd like the body opened. Peters then turned to Paul and said, "Scrub and begin. I have one or

two things to take care of, but I'll be back to help you." Paul scrubbed, prepared and draped the body, and began the operation. Peters never returned. Paul began to grumble as he did the procedure. A few times he asked the scrub nurse for instructions: What type of suture was normally used? How big an incision should he make to bring the colostomy out? How much bowel should he exteriorize? and so on. As soon as the procedure was finished, he sought out Able's chief resident, Mark, and complained: "Listen, if I had known Peters wasn't coming back, I would never have done that alone. I didn't know what I was doing." Mark did what he could to calm Paul, who was very upset. Mark kept pointing out how well the operation had gone. Paul remained unconvinced (Able Service).

Such breaches are, however, rare; and it is these exceptions and the strong feelings that they mobilize that allow us to infer how much a tightly controlled, well-supervised division of labor is the norm.

A more common problem is the reverse situation: beginning housestaff feel that the training process moves too slowly and that they are not getting enough experience or enough opportunity to exercise their judgment:

In the dinner line this evening, Brian, an intern, was complaining to Josh, a second-year resident, about doing a breast biopsy with Ernest, Baker's chief resident. Brian said, "I lost my biopsy to Ernest today." Josh asked, "What do you mean? Didn't he let you do it?" Brian answered, "Yeah, he let me do it. But he's real intrusive to work with. He couldn't keep his hands out of my operative field. If that ever happens again, I'll refuse to scrub with him again" (Baker Service).

The threat is idle, but the complaint is real. We should be alert to the fact that when this incident occurred Brian had been an intern only a month, yet he already felt the control of work confining. Another event a few days later further illustrates the point:

After rounds, Ernest broke off from the rest of the Baker Service and went to the outpatient department to do a biopsy. After he left, a junior student asked where he had gone. Brian answered, "To do a junior student case." He then turned to me and went on without prompting, "Ernest takes a lot of cases that a chief resident has no business touching. Cases that Josh and I should be doing. It's really frustrating—he just grabs up everything." I asked Brian why Ernest would do this. He responded, "It's because Arthur and Grant do things that you just don't expect attendings to touch. So Ernest never feels he has enough to do. So he takes cases from Josh and then Josh takes cases from me. It's all very frustrating" (Baker Service).

The argot of a surgery service associates operative problems with rank: a "junior student case" is a simple procedure, one for the most untrained; and an "attending case" is the most difficult of procedures. To accuse the chief resident of doing junior student cases is therefore to make a serious complaint about the division of labor and responsibility. Nevertheless, what is at issue here is not whether the two attendings hogged cases; on the same service at the end of the previous training year, there were no complaints about the division of labor. Control of work and supervision is most intense during the early stages of the training year and relaxes as training proceeds and subordinates gain exposure to and experience with new techniques. We should not be surprised that the graduates of elite medical schools find a rigid division of labor frustrating, but neither should we overlook how this division of labor serves to minimize technical error.

A second factor is operative on surgical services which also serves to suppress the absolute number of technical errors: namely, all requests for help are viewed as legitimate. When instructions for tasks are given, they are invariably followed by the tag line, "If you run into any problems, give me a call." This statement is more than conversational filler; it is a reminder to subordinates that their superordinates are legally responsible for their actions and are available to help. Further, the statement passes on to the subordinate the responsibility of seeking help in situations beyond his level of competence. An important part of the subordinate's training is learning to discriminate between situations which he can and cannot handle. A request for aid is always honored. Two superordinate responses are common: (1) either the next person in the hierarchy performs the task himself, or (2) verbal instructions or pointers are offered. The first option is exercised when either time demands quick performance of the task, or when the task itself is seen as more complex than previously imagined:

> A myleogram [a diagnostic procedure involving the removal of spinal fluid and the injection of dye in the spinal column] was ordered for Mr. Eckhardt. A senior student was to instruct a junior student in the procedure. They tried without any success to get the needle in the proper space. After some fumbling and a few sticks at Eckhardt the senior student instructed the junior student to "get Paul." Paul came in and surveyed the situation. After examining Eckhardt's back he told the students, who were profusely apologizing for their failure, not to worry; that the problem was in Mr. Eckhardt's anatomy and not in their skills. He then proceeded with some difficulty to complete the procedure, instructing the students all the while (Able Service).

The skill of housestaff with such procedures helps establish their authority to students. The ease with which they place intravenous needles in the veins of the most troublesome patients is a very common way to impress students; it serves especially to humble senior students who are planning surgical careers and who are often competitive with first-year housestaff. The second option, verbal instructions and pointers, is exercised when, in the judgment of the superordinate, the task is not beyond the skill of the subordinate but rather the individual's lack of confidence in his own abilities is preventing task performance. Here, the subordinate is made to see that he can accomplish the task and at the same time he is offered support. Surgical housestaff learn to operate in much the same way that small children learn to ride bicycles. An unseen hand supports their efforts. The hand is withdrawn by stages and the novice finds himself operating on his own:

> Carl, the intern, was closing an incision while Mark, the chief resident, was assisting. Carl was ill at ease. He turned to Mark and said, "I can't do it." Mark said, "What do you mean, you can't? Don't ever say you can't. Of course you can." "No, I just can't seem to get it right." Carl had been forced to put in and remove stitches a number of times, unable to draw the skin closed with the proper tension. Mark replied, "Really, there's nothing to it"; and, taking Carl's hand in his own, he said, "The trick is to keep the needle at this angle and put the stitch through like this," all the while leading Carl through the task. "Now, go on." Mark then let Carl struggle through the rest of the closure on his own (Able Service).

Technical errors, then, are distributed throughout the surgical division of labor, but unevenly. More are made by beginners than the experienced. Technical errors do not damage an individual's claims to competence so long as he appears to learn from them and to make less of them over time. Supervision and the division of labor are arranged to keep such errors at a minimum.

Judgmental Errors

A judgmental error occurs when an incorrect strategy of treatment is chosen. These errors are also unevenly distributed through the division of labor. Subordinates who have only little discretionary power make few and relatively minor judgmental errors. Attending surgeons in charge of devising treatment plans make the most and the most serious judgmental errors. In these cases judgment is not always incorrect in any absolute sense; the surgeon, given the clinical evidence available at the time, may have chosen an eminently reasonable course of action, but the result—a death or complication—forces the surgeon to consider whether some alternative might have been more profitably employed. Clinical results, not scientific reasoning, determine how correct judgment is. Surgeons have an aphorism that expresses this: "Excellent surgery makes dead patients." By this they state most flat-footedly their understanding that textbook principles of care have to be compromised to meet the immediate situation, that results and not the elegance of a clinical blueprint separate acceptable from unacceptable practice.

The two most common judgmental errors that attendings make are (1) overly heroic surgery, and (2) the failure to operate when the situation demands. Overly heroic surgery involves the decision to operate when the patient cannot tolerate the procedure. This decision to operate is a surgeon's commitment to his skills; it is also a moral-ethical decision about what "tolerable" risk is and a decision about what the proper role of the physician is—whether he is charged with merely sustaining life or whether he may subject his patients to great risk in order to upgrade the quality of life. Needless to say, these are not easy or pleasant decisions. Consider the following:

> Mrs. Hardy is an old patient of Dr. Peters who has metastatic cancer. She has at most a few months to live. Recently her condition has worsened. Without an operation, she will probably literally vomit to death within a month. She has poor pulmonary and cardiac function; it is not clear whether she could tolerate an operation. If one is successfully performed, her life expectancy would be between three and six months— a month and a half of which would be postoperative convalescence (Able Service).

In this case can the surgeon justify putting a patient through the risk and trauma of surgery for such dubious rewards? But in good conscience can he stand idly by and sentence her to such an unpleasant death? An attending makes these decisions for him-self. He may ask his subordinates what they would do if the decision were theirs. A favorite way of phrasing this question is, "What would you do if the patient were your mother?" After listening to his subordinates, the attending announces his de-cision. He need not justify this choice to other attendings. He need not explain the basis of his decision to his subordinates, although the didactic situation of surgical training encourages such explanations. To mobilize the resources necessary for action, the attending need only make up his mind. In this sense, his patients are his to do with as he wishes.

If subordinates disagree with an attending, there is very little they can do. A common tactic is to anticipate complications from a procedure and ask the attending how he intends to manage them:

Mrs. Pratt is an obese woman with metastatic cancer on whom Dr. White has decided to perform an adrenalectomy and an oophorectomy [surgical removal of adrenal glands and the ovaries; an attempt to achieve a remission from cancer]. Mrs. Pratt's obesity and very poor pulmonary function make her a very poor operative risk. Both Mark and Paul seemed uneasy with White's decision. Mark told White that Mrs. Pratt would be like "a beached whale" following surgery and then he asked White a series of questions about the possibilities of embolism and the prophylactic measures White had in mind and about the difficulties of managing her pulmonary status following surgery. Paul then asked about gallstones and the possibilities of cholecystitis [inflammation of gallbladder]. After answering these objections, White left. Paul and Mark confided to each other that they felt uneasy about the surgery. Neither was certain that they would recommend it for their mother. Later, when I told Paul he seemed uncomfortable about the decision to operate, he replied: "Well, there is a great risk involved and it's not clear to me that the benefits are greater than chemotherapy, although White is right—the results of surgery can be absolutely dramatic, if you are lucky. Look—it's one thing for a patient to die from disease; you don't like it, but there's nothing you can do about it; you accept it. But for a patient to die because of something you did to him, because you gave him pulmonary edema [filling of lungs with fluid], or from a leaking anastomosis [seams that join resected body parts], that's a whole different thing. It makes you feel real bad when something you did kills somebody. It gives you pause for thought. Doctors aren't supposed to do that" (Able Service).

However, no matter how much they disagree with an attending's decision, no matter how much they grumble among themselves, subordinates defer to decisions with no more than polite questioning. The decision to operate is an apparently unchallengeable element in an attending's professional autonomy:

> I just make it a point not to disagree with attendings for two reasons. First, I'm not as smart as they are. And, second, the ultimate responsibility is theirs; and if they think that something should be done, I'll do it (Intern).

A second common judgmental error of attendings is the failure to establish a clear-cut plan of action for chronic problems. For most of these patients, secondary problems make operating impossible. These patients tend to linger in the hospital. They are not discharged nor are they aggressively treated. Often diagnostic tests reveal conditions in addition to the original problem requiring hospitalization. Each test in turn requires a further one. Intensive diagnostic studies are done on the patient even though he will not be extensively treated:

> Surgeons in general don't like theoretical or psychological problems. Things are either black or white. If they don't understand something, they try to put it out of their minds. For example, there are two patients on our service now whom we can't do anything with, and they really need something done. I think they will die without operations. But they are too sick to be operated on. The surgeon in this case gets frustrated and less aggressive. One of the worst things that can happen to a patient is to spend a long time on a surgical service. Surgeons lose interest in chronic problems. When the surgeon begins to lose interest, he starts asking for consultations, hoping that someone will take responsibility for the patient. Unfortunately some patients, not a lot, die because the surgeon loses interest (Chief Resident).

The error in judgment here need not express itself in a death or complication; surgical patients can spend considerable periods of time in the hospital, have little done for them, and be discharged without incident. Nevertheless, precious healing resources have been misallocated—a bed is taken up, time and effort are expended, and what the surgeon hoped to accomplish for the patient is never made certain. Moreover, such mistakes are more

likely to be overlooked than others because they are not marked
by an objective event such as death.

Though judgmental errors are most commonly made by attendings, some are also made by housestaff who have to make immediate decisions about patient management:

> Sam Jerome had his appendix removed on Baker Service. His
> postoperative recovery was anything but smooth. He was
> reoperated on for what was diagnosed as an obstruction but
> turned out to be an ileus [a condition where bowel has no
> peristaltic action]. Following the second operation, he
> developed a wound infection. Two days after the second
> operation, Brian, an intern, was sitting in the Baker confer-
> ence room. I asked him how it was going and he replied, "Not
> so good. This responsibility can be devastating. It's just
> awesome. Take Jerome—I couldn't help thinking that the
> phenobarbital I ordered for him postop may have given him
> the ileus that caused us to think he was obstructed. That made
> us reoperate, and then he gets this wound infection"
> (Baker Service).

Housestaff routinely make such self-criticisms of their behavior, especially after deaths and complications. They review their
entire course of action to see where they might have acted differently. Attendings encourage this reexamination of action and see
it as symbolic of a subordinate's determination to learn:

> Until he is confident and secure, any good surgeon dreams
> about his operations. He reoperates, taking stitches in and
> out, revising his approach. He does this, too, for clinical
> situations. He rethinks how each patient was managed. This
> happens until he's secure. I did it. I expect my housestaff to
> do it. You need this kind of attention to detail, absolute
> dedication, and personal honesty to be a good surgeon
> (Attending).

Despite their claims of making serious and consequential judgmental errors, housestaff are not sanctioned for them for a number of reasons. First, they do not have the responsibility to make
serious judgmental decisions; and, as Stelling and Bucher (1972)
have shown for psychiatric and medical wards, one cannot be

accountable for an event unless one is also responsible for it. Second, like technical errors, when quickly reported and infrequently committed, judgmental errors are seen as an inevitable cost of training. They do not indicate that an individual is incompetent but rather they serve as evidence that he needs further teaching. Judgmental errors, then, also reinforce a "training" definition of the situation. Furthermore, as we shall see in chapter 4, there are structural limits placed on the housestaff's ability to indulge in self-criticism. While social control of action rests on self-criticism, the process of self-criticism itself is subject to social controls.

Attendings are also somewhat insulated from the negative implications of their judgmental errors. First, their professional accomplishments protect them from the imputation of defective judgment: any individual failure must be weighed against many successes, research publications, and the like. Second, operating on difficult cases that others would not handle is a pride of place. The attendings at Pacific pride themselves on their ability to treat such cases. Death from judgmental error in such trying situations is an uncomfortable fact of life:

> It would look suspicious if you are doing major surgery and, week after week, you have no deaths and complications. You're going to have these, especially deaths, if you do major surgery. You can lead a long and happy life without deaths and complications, but you have to give up major surgery (Attending).

There are times then when the surgical expectation of success is waived. The reputation of the individual attendings of the surgery department at Pacific and the reputation of the department itself encourages heroic surgery in risky situations. In these cases, some judgmental error is expected. These are not severely judged. Such cases are seen not so much as mistakes but as a privilege and as a burden of rank. Judgmental error in heroic situations—or operating too often in heroic situations—may earn an attending a reputation among his colleagues and subordinates as a "matador," a "gunslinger," or "someone who sees a patient as just so much meat on a table." Yet while such terms are indicative that the attending is not held in high esteem by his colleagues, being so labeled seems to have no noticeable effect on day-to-day behavior. It should also be noted that as a term of opprobrium there is a certain ambivalence involved in calling someone a "gunslinger" or a "matador." After all, in their respective cultures, such figures symbolize the heroic ideal. I suspect that most surgeons would rather be compared to Wild Bill Hickcock or Billy the Kid than to Caspar Milquetoast or Walter Mitty.

Normative Errors

A normative error occurs when a surgeon has, in the eyes of others, failed to discharge his role obligations conscientiously. Technical and judgmental errors are errors in a role; normative errors signal error in assuming a role. These errors are not distributed throughout the division of labor but are almost exclusively subordinate errors. Normative error occurs when, in the attending's judgment, a houseofficer's conduct violates the working understandings on which action rests. When a normative error occurs, the mistake renders it impossible to consider the person making it—in legal terms—a just and reasonably prudent individual. Viewed sociologically, normative errors challenge tacit background assumptions about how reality in a scene is constructed.

When spelled out, the background assumptions that govern clinical action are few, and they are drilled into the subordinate from his first clinical rotation as a medical student. The covering law for all behavior is, simply stated, "No surprises." Superordinates expect their subordinates to inform them of all changes, however small, in the service's status:

> During the orientation meeting for the Able Service, Mark, the chief resident, explained what he expected during the next rotation: "If anything comes up, I want to know about it. I don't care what time it is; I want you to call. If there is a problem at four in the morning call at four in the morning.

Most likely, I'll listen to what you tell me and fall right back to sleep. I may even forget that you called. But call. I don't like to walk in here in the morning and find myself surprised by what's going on in my service. I'm ultimately responsible for what goes on here, so call me." He repeated this message a number of times in a number of ways (Able Service).

The no-surprises rule is shared by all attendings. When interviewed, they all stated that the first expectation for housestaff performance is compliance with the rule of no surprises. Interpreting the no-surprises edict is in actual practice a complex decision for housestaff. Attendings dogmatically state the rule to impress housestaff with its importance and to rescue everyone from the technical and judgmental errors that are part of being inexpert. Nevertheless, whether or not in any particular instance to invoke the rule and call is a recurrent problem for subordinates. On the one hand, the housestaff member does not want to look foolish, as if he cannot handle the simplest situations; and on the other, he does not want to risk the attending's anger or the patient's life should his assessment of the situation be incorrect. Perhaps it needs to be pointed out that when a subordinate chooses not to invoke the rule and does not call, he still risks the attending's wrath even if he acts in a technically correct fashion. At no time did I observe superordinates reacting negatively to subordinates who called them for what later became unnecessary reasons; and often what appears at the time as an unnecessary reason appears retrospectively as very consequential:

Don, the senior student, at the end of a long and an eventful day—there had been one unexpected death and one kidney transplant—was talking with Greg, a junior student. "I called Mark last night about Thelma Halsted [the unexpected death]. It was four in the morning and he wasn't too pleased. He told me to do what I would have done anyway. But the way things worked out today, I'm really glad I called" (Able Service).

Idealists may be dismayed that Don's reaction to an unexpected death is relief that he cannot be blamed. The more hard-

boiled and pragmatic will be grateful that from a personal tragedy, a moral lesson was salvaged and reinforced: when in doubt,
call, lest a death be your undoing. For the subordinate, calling is
always a safe strategy. Interpreting the no-surprises rule in the
framework of a zero-sum two-person game, a subordinate always
makes a game-correct decision to call. Yet subordinates feel that
there are costs attached to calling and may be under great pressure not to call because more than a correct response in an
interaction game is involved. In addition to the fear of looking
foolish, there is the desire to participate early in the intrinsic
gratifications of surgery, the belief that one learns from managing
new clinical situations, and a sense of dedication to the heroic
ideal that one is made or unmade by the quality of one's tests:

> The way you learn as an intern is by being put on the spot and
> coming through it. You develop a self-awareness that you can
> handle a lot of situations. The problem is learning what situa-
> tions you can't handle. There's a lot of pressure not to ask,
> a lot of fear of appearing foolish (Intern).

Despite these tensions and the resulting temptation for the subordinate to go it on his own, the no-surprises rule is the overarching
principle by which normative errors are defined.

We may ask, What is a surprise? The most correct answer is
anything that an attending chooses; and even though housestaff
occasionally feel that attendings apply no principles of selection,
attending behavior is more predictable than that. First, a surprise
for an attending is any violation of the principle of full and honest
disclosure. A surprise for the attending carries with it the implication that a housestaff member was lazy, negligent, or dishonest.
In practical terms, an attending finds himself surprised when he
discovers for himself something about a patient that housestaff
knew and neglected to tell him, or when he discovers for himself
something his housestaff should have known:

> I walked into the intensive care unit with Carl, Able's
> resident. Dr. White was on the phone. "I see a glucose value
> of 540," he grunts, and screws his face in an expression of
> pain. "Well, we were planning to operate today, but obviously

we've changed our thinking." White hung up and asked,
"What's this I hear about Thelma Halsted?" "I'm just getting
the story myself, sir," Paul, a second-year resident, answered.
"She had to be rushed to the Cardiac Care Unit for a pace-
maker. She's doing terribly," Carl volunteered. "Carl, why
wasn't I told?" Carl: "You were operating on the transplant,
sir." White: "That's no excuse. If you couldn't get away, you
could have called up to the OR and they would have tacked a
note on the door that I would have gotten the minute I
finished the case. That way, after surgery, I wouldn't stop
for coffee. I wouldn't stop and talk to people. Listen—when
one of my patients is dying, I don't like to be told by some
damn medical intern. I want to know what's going on with my
patients." White then wadded a piece of paper and threw it
across the nurses' station (Able Service).

Dr. Arthur was concerned that a complication from the
operation on Mrs. Prewitt might be a perineal nerve palsy
[temporary paralysis of the foot from operative damage to the
perineal nerve]. In clinic when he asked Ernest, the chief
resident, and Josh, the second-year resident, about it, they
both assured him that on morning rounds she was quite all
right. However, her examination on afternoon rounds revealed
a perineal nerve palsy. Dr. Arthur's anger was apparent as we
left the room. We walked about sixty feet down the corridor
before he stopped to speak: "Goddammit! I will not have this
on my service. Do you understand? I ask if the patient has a
perineal nerve palsy and am assured by my housestaff that
she doesn't and she damn well does. Now, this is not caused
by your not being smart enough to recognize the problem. It's
not your skill that is wanting here. This is a case pure and
simple of your being too lazy to get off your asses and look at
the patients. I will not tolerate this. Did you see this patient
this morning, Ernest?" "I did—yes, I did, sir." Arthur: "And
you didn't notice that she had no dorsal flexion [movement of
the foot at the ankle]?" Ernest: "No, sir." "Well, what the
hell were you looking at? What am I going to have to do to
get this service running right? If I can't count on my housestaff to provide decent preoperative and postoperative care
for my patients, then Grant and I will cancel our operations

until the patients we have are under control and until we are sure that we have housestaff who can do the job. Do I make myself clear?'' (Baker Service).

Normative breaches are breaches of the etiquette governing the role relations between attending surgeons and housestaff. A normative error in turn carries with it the implication that a fundamental breach of etiquette governing the role relation between doctor and patient has occurred. When making decisions, the surgeon—any physician, in fact—is expected to bracket all systems of relevance to him as an actor in his other social roles and even bracket all systems of relevance to him in his other capacities as a surgeon. He is expected to treat conditions as they arise or to make certain that they will be treated before he moves on to other tasks. Fatigue, pressing family problems, a long queue of patients waiting to be seen, a touch of the flu—all the excuses that individuals routinely use in everyday life, are inadmissible on a surgery service. An attending who is surprised assumes that his housestaff have not been dispensing proper clinical care. Had they been, housestaff would have informed him of changes in clinical status.

Attendings are most frequently surprised by housestaff not keeping them abreast of unfolding events, but there are two other types of surprises that are treated as normative errors. A housestaff member's inability to get along with nurses is a failure that attendings treat as normative. It violates the tacit assumption that one will not let personality intrude on clinical care:

After rounds, Arthur turned to Sharon, the head nurse of Baker Service, and asked: "Are there any nursing problems?" "Plenty!" Sharon replied. At Arthur's suggestion, we all went into the conference room to discuss it. Sharon explained that Dr. Carter and the nurses "didn't seem to get along this weekend." Arthur turned to Carter: "All right, Carter—what's the problem?" Carter explained: "Well, we had some problems getting a urinalysis done on Mrs. Yardley. The urine was collected but no one took it to the General Services Lab until I did at midnight. That's just one thing, but, really, the nurses on this floor are incredible. All the housestaff have complained about it. The other night I was called every fifteen minutes. Once I was called because Crane's IV wasn't running. When I came down, I saw he had rolled over and kinked it. It was obvious that the night staff hadn't even looked at it." Arthur answered: "None of that bothers me. If you have to get up every fifteen minutes because nurses are too tired, lazy, or stupid, that's too bad for you, but it's what you're paid to do. You may even lose a pound or two. [Carter is overweight.] What bothers me is your fighting with staff. That accomplished nothing. In fact, it makes things worse. Look—you're a professional, you are better educated, better trained, and supposedly more mature than the staff. If you can't get along with them, we'll find someone who can. Do I make myself clear?" (Baker Service).

Housestaff failure to maintain good working relations on the ward is a serious mistake; it indicates that a subordinate lacks the skills necessary to run a surgical team. A housestaff member who quarrels with support staff is blamed—whatever the legitimacy of his complaint—for placing his own needs above those of patient care. There are ways of dealing with improper nursing; public quarreling is not among them. Further, as far as an attending is concerned, the problem with a subordinate who quarrels with nurses because they call too often for unnecessary reasons is that when he becomes a chief resident he may complain about his interns and that when he becomes an attending he may complain about his chief residents. This complaining may communicate that he is unavailable to help. In this case the whole set of controls built into task performance by the division of labor and norms of clinical care breaks down. Complaints about unnecessary work indicate to superordinates that a subordinate lacks the proper commitment.

A second serious error is similar to inability to work agreeably with nurses, that is, the inability to secure the cooperation of patients and their families. To housestaff fall the problems of obtaining informed consent, of gaining the patient's cooperation for preoperative and postoperative care—this is especially important because the involved patient can do much to prevent some postoperative complications, and of managing the anxieties of the patient and his family. A failure at any of these tasks is an indication that a subordinate cannot control the normal troubles of his environment. In addition, failure at any of these tasks creates extra work for attendings—these are unpleasant surprises—and all of this work is considered avoidable. It all stems from a subordinate not conscientiously filling his role. Technical and judgmental errors also create extra work, but such work is seen as an inevitable part of surgery. However, the extra work of normative errors is unnecessary. It is not viewed as an inevitable part of major surgery but as an inevitable consequence of minor surgeons.

Although normative errors are committed by both subordinates and superordinates, only those of housestaff are criticized and punished. Housestaff make normative errors because they are subject to so many cross-cutting systems of relevance that it is often impossible for them to bracket all systems of relevance, keep unfolding action under control, and avoid unnecessary problems for attendings. An intern or second-year resident's schedule is a grueling one: he works six and a half days, fifty weeks a year; a light working day is twelve hours; and at least two nights a week he stays in the hospital on call for emergencies. Given such working conditions, many other systems of relevance impose on the clinical one. There is the physiological one: housestaff need to eat and sleep. There is the social one: housestaff need time-out periods (this is an especially acute problem for married housestaff). There is the student one: housestaff need to study the problems they are treating. All of these are in addition to the multiple systems of the clinical role itself, which requires housestaff to coordinate treatment for as many as thirty-five patients, to provide a full complement of ancillary services, and to keep the ward running smoothly. Undoubtedly, trying to meet such multifocal demands explains to some degree why normative error occurs. Attendings, however, never allow such factors to excuse normative error. For them, there is no "good" excuse for a normative error because no other system of relevance is ever allowed ascendancy over the basic doctor-patient dyad and because normative errors are always interpreted as evidence that the houseofficer placed some other concern above patient care.

This is so despite the fact that normative errors such as quarrels with nurses or the failure to keep attendings fully informed need not result in outcomes that directly harm the patient. On the other hand, technical and judgmental errors always involve some discomfort to the patient yet are often interpreted as evidence of the individual houseofficer's commitment to clinical care.

Attendings escape blame for their normative errors for three reasons. First, the privileges of rank insulate them from many of the housestaff's cross-pressures. Because of their rank they are directly accountable to no one on a day-to-day basis. Second, membership in the American College of Surgeons, appointment to the Pacific faculty, and other credentials such as research publications and professional awards are a presumptive moral licensing. To be an attending at Pacific is to stand at the symbolic center of the value system of American medicine.[5] Basically, an attending is not publicly blamed for normative errors because there is no one to accuse him of such moral lapses. No one stands above him in the hierarchy and enforces the rule of "no surprises." The attending's position contrasts sharply with that of the houseofficer who has not yet been certified as morally fit to be a surgeon, whose commitments are now being tested. Third, although the attending is the legally responsible agent for patient care, the division of labor does not always reflect this. Generally attendings spend the greater portion of their time teaching or doing research rather than providing direct clinical care. Housestaff spend virtually all of their time providing direct care. Thus, division of labor itself frees the attending from the more prosaic responsibilities and pressures of patient care. All of these fall to housestaff, a fact which exposes them to concrete charges of normative failure. Rank, moral authority, and everyday task-structure insulate the attending and expose the housestaff to the danger of normative error.

Normative errors are taken seriously by housestaff and attendings. Housestaff fear normative error much more than they do technical and judgmental errors. They fear that normative errors destroy their credibility as responsible workers; they fear bad recommendations and other negative sanctions:

After he failed to inform Dr. White of Thelma Halsted's deteriorating condition and after White had reprimanded him, Carl left the room and sat dejected on a bench. He said: "That's it. I just blew two months' hard work in two minutes. It doesn't matter now what my work on the service was like. This is all he'll remember. It was a really dumb thing to do, a serious faux pas. I don't think she would have had any different care, really there was nothing White could have done about it. I guess it's just embarrassing for him to have a resident from another service tell him about his patients" (Able Service).

This fear of normative error on the part of housestaff runs deep and is shared by medical students. Among the students, we can see more clearly the logic-in-use that develops around performance and failure. Junior and senior medical students often state that the tasks they are assigned are so minor as to be worthless in evaluating their clinical skills. As a result, they think evaluations are based on their ability to be team members. Like housestaff, they are frightened of receiving recommendations that brand them as individuals who have difficulty respecting proper lines of authority. Interns and students both suffer the less rewarding aspects of their position in silence for fear of the repercussions of an overly noisy complaint:

Irv and Larry, the two students on Baker, have been dissatisfied with their stay on the service and were vigorously complaining to Christian, the intern, about it. Irv said: "It's not the amount of work, Chris—it's what we learn from it. We are not learning the principles of surgery and that's why we are here. What are we going to learn from anyway: doing the scut work or working-up a few patients and following through on them and reading about their problems?" Larry added: "Yeah, I don't mind being on call with the service because then you learn something. You work-up patients and see things. But to stay at the hospital just to change IV's—that doesn't make any sense." Chris answered: "Look—I didn't arrange the way that the service runs. If you have such complaints, if you feel this way, you should talk to Dr. Grant or Dr. Arthur." Irv replied: "C'mon, Chris. You know that we can't do that. We don't want a recommendation that says the student is unmotivated, uninterested in patients, and hard to work with. We want to work with patients, but we want to learn something, too" (Baker Service).

Attending reaction to normative error justifies housestaff's fear of these breaches. Attendings react strongly to normative error for a number of reasons. First, in the early stages of training, there are only minor variations in skill among subordinates. Normative performance is seen as an indicator of honesty and responsibility, two qualities that attendings feel subordinates must possess if they are to be capable colleagues:

> The most important thing is complete intellectual honesty, a willingness to admit problems and personal deficiencies. Someone who recognizes his errors and 'fesses up.' Look, I could teach a gorilla to operate in six months, but I can't teach honesty and responsibility. It's the people who have these qualities who make outstanding surgeons (Attending).

A technical or judgmental error then says something to an attending about a recruit's level of training; a normative error says something about the recruit himself. A second reason that normative breaches are so serious is that patients for whom attendings are legally responsible can be lost, without the attending's best effort being made on their behalf. A normative error then compounds the normal troubles of a surgeon's life. In addition to the inevitable deaths and complications, he must worry with those caused by personal as opposed to professional shortcomings; he is dealing with reducible error:

> Covering up is never really excusable. You have to remember that each time a resident hides information, he is affecting someone's life. Now in this business it takes a lot of self-confidence, a lot of maturity, to admit errors. But that's not the issue. No mistakes are minor. All have a mortality and a morbidity. Say I have a patient who comes back from the operating room and he doesn't urinate. And say my intern doesn't notice or he decides it's nothing serious and he doesn't catheterize the guy and he doesn't tell me. Well, this guy's bladder

fills up. There's a foreign body and foreign bodies can cause infections; infection can become sepsis; sepsis can cause death. So the intern's mistake here can cause this guy hundreds of dollars in extra hospitalization and it could cost him his life. All mistakes have costs attached to them. Now a certain amount are inevitable. But it is the obligation of everyone involved in patient care to minimize mistakes. The way to do that is by full and total disclosure (Attending).

A normative error breaches this system of full and open disclosure: this system protects attendings at the same time that it frees them for other activities. They need not be omnipresent if their housestaff keep them omniscient. The subordinate who fails here can expect severe punishments.[6] The rule of thumb attendings apply here is, even the most technically incompetent can be trained for something—he will rise or sink to his own level of proficiency. But the morally bankrupt represents a threat to the surgeons at Pacific and must be treated as a serious problem.

Quasi-normative Errors

Normative errors are breaches of standards of performance that all attendings share: quasi-normative errors are eccentric and attending-specific. Each attending has certain protocols that he and he alone follows. A subordinate who does not follow these rules mocks his superordinate's authority; his behavior is a claim that his judgment is as adequate as his superior's; and even though in no absolute sense can one claim that a mistake has been made, a subordinate who makes a quasi-normative error risks his reputation as a trustworthy recruit.

There are many decisions which surgeons are forced to make in the absence of scientifically established criteria. Great uncertainty surrounds much medical behavior.[7] From their own clinical experience and from medical journals, attendings marshal evidence to support one approach to a particular problem as opposed to another. However, the evidence is far from conclusive, debate continues, and a consensus fails to emerge. Some attendings approach a problem in one fashion with very good results;

others have equally good results with a competing approach. Despite the open-ended nature of the question "Which approach is better?", attendings in their everyday behavior can be quite dogmatic. Attendings believe that housestaff are on *their* services to learn *their* approach to the surgical management of disease. On other services, they can learn *other* approaches. Nevertheless, attendings are quite capable of making the theoretic distinction that separates quasi-normative from genuine error:

> First, you have to recognize that there are two different types of mistakes. There are genuine mistakes and there are mistakes of the "I don't do it this way; do it my way" variety. Those really aren't mistakes. At this hospital, for instance, take a patient with gastrointestinal bleeding. If he enters Dr. Arthur's service, Arthur wants to locate the source of bleeding. He performs an endoscopy [a procedure to view an internal organ; in this case the stomach is viewed through the mouth] on the patient, takes X rays, and maybe does an angiogram to locate the source of bleeding. Now, Dr. Henry doesn't think it's important to locate the source of bleeding. He places a nasogastric tube down the patient to suction any clots and get the stomach free of blood; he milks the stomach with an antacid bath; and if the bleeding stops, he doesn't care about the source. He figures if the bleeding doesn't stop, he still has time to do the tests to locate the source. One approaches the problem conservatively; the other, radically. Now these are both tremendously prominent men in the field. Who is to say that one way is right and the other is a mistake? (Attending).

In any actual case, the attending who is responsible for the patient's care is the one who says whether one approach is correct or not. The subordinate who favors and initiates another attending's approach over the one on whose service he is working opens himself up to severe criticism:

> On rounds, Dr. Arthur was examining the incision of Mrs. Anders, a young woman who had just received her second mastectomy. After reassuring her that everything was fine, everyone left her room. We walked a bit down the hall and Arthur exploded: "That wound looks like a walking piece of

dogshit. We don't close wounds with continuous suture on
this service. We worked for hours giving this lady the best
possible operation and then you screw it up on the closure.
That's not how we close wounds on this service, understand?
These are the fine points that separate good surgeons from
butchers, and that's what you are here to learn. I never want
to see another wound closed like that. Never!" Arthur then
was silent, he walked a few feet, and then he began speaking
again: "I don't give a shit how Dr. Henry does it on the
Charlie Service or how Dr. Gray does it on Dogface; when
you're on my service, you'll do it the way I want. There's
no excuse for this, especially after I gave a little speech at
Thursday's conference that I never use continuous sutures. If
you work for me, you do things my way. I don't want any
work screwed up by incompetent closures. Do you understand?" (Baker Service).

For the attending, more than professional pride is involved in
quasi-normative errors: housestaff using their own independent
judgment appear insubordinate to him. Compliance with attending dictates, however open to debate they are, is an indicator that
a subordinate is a responsible member of the team who can be
trusted. Attendings feel that the subordinate who makes quasi-
normative errors is also likely to make normative errors: his
behavior does not inspire trust:

The thing that offends me the most is when I tell someone
they made a mistake and I give him my list of reasons—
because he's always entitled to know why he is wrong—and
then he tells me that it was okay, and that he was entitled to
make a mistake for his own experience. When people put
their own experience above patient care, I find it intolerable.
Just the other day, I had a fourth-year student pull a nasogastric tube on the second day postop of a patient of mine. I
told him that this was not wise. The patient had no bowel
sounds nor had he had a bowel movement, and I take both as
indications that a nasogastric tube is ready to be pulled—
however, in this guy's judgment what he did was okay. He
ignored my reasons. In fact, this guy's goal was not to be
responsible for patient care but to be independent of higher-

ups. He told me what he did was important for his own clinical development. He didn't give a fig about patient care. And nothing—nothing—nixes my confidence quicker than that. It's a privilege to learn here and the student is obligated to have a respect for our methods. They have to respect that the responsibility for the patient is ours; it's not the resident's patient—it's ours (Attending).

When a normative breach is made, a double error is involved: standards of clinical care are breached and the etiquette governing role relations among attendings and housestaff is breached. For quasi-normative errors, clinical care may be correctly administered and the general etiquette of role relations may even be followed—the subordinate may have informed his superior of the problem and been told to take care of it in the "usual" way. When a quasi-normative error is made, the subordinate is wrong for all the right reasons: his fault is that of *hubris*: he tried to act like an attending. Quasi-normative errors are idiosyncratic; behavior that would be formally correct on one service is not so on another. This is the cutting edge that distinguishes normative from quasi-normative errors: what counts as a normative breach is fairly constant from service to service. Nevertheless, attendings recognize each other's right to organize and run their services as they see fit; they hold that it is the subordinate's responsibility to accommodate himself to this state of affairs; and they agree that quasi-normative errors indicate that something is seriously awry with a subordinate.

The organization of work on a service determines how much room a subordinate will have for independent judgment and consequently how likely it is that he will make quasi-normative errors. On the Able Service, where supervision is relatively loose, subordinates have a great deal of room to maneuver and quasi-normative errors are relatively rare occurrences. On the Baker Service, supervision is relatively tight, subordinates have little room, and quasi-normative errors are more common. Housestaff when on the Baker Service state that they have to be "company men." Dr. Arthur has numerous personal eccentricities which he expects housestaff to respect and learn from. These express themselves in various eponyms: there are Arthur variations of operative procedures; there is the Arthur fluid-management regimen for postop care; and there is the Arthur method for managing gastrointestinal bleeding. Given the autocratic nature of surgical authority, the strong personal preferences of superiors are translated into absolute rules of conduct for subordinates. In everyday life, we label those with this power prima donnas: their own likes and dislikes become the rules others follow.

For their part, housestaff are eager to avoid quasi-normative errors. They fear finding themselves on an attending's wrong side, a state of affairs which can have devastating effects given the amount of control that attendings have over their careers. Often, the steps subordinates take to avoid quasi-normative errors can be amusing to the observer and sufficiently detached participant:

> Mark, Baker's chief resident, and Stan, a third-year resident, walked into Mr. Johnson's room on morning rounds. "Oh, my God! What's this?" they said in unison. "That's the patient with gastrointestinal bleeding I called you about last night," said John, the intern. "But you're treating him with an antacid bath," Stan said. "Sure! Isn't that the usual treatment? It's the way Henry does it on Charlie," said John. "You never treat gastrointestinal bleeding that way on Arthur's service. He'll blow his top if he sees this. We better get this out of here quickly," said Stan, all the while removing the antacid bath. As we left the room, Mark turned to me and said that a lot of surgery was foolishness and a lot of what surgeons believed was magic. But you couldn't argue with results (Baker Service).

More commonly, housestaff are not good-natured about meeting what seem to them the mere whims of superordinates; quasi-normative errors are a source of tension among housestaff and attendings. Housestaff resent that their judgment is not trusted; they feel that they are not given tasks commensurate with their skills; and they feel exploited as a cheap source of labor. Especially vexing to housestaff is the lack of debate and questioning that precedes many decisions:

I don't like it when orders are given down from above without reasoning. I do not like decisions when there is no discussion. I realize that questions are not always appropriate; but when they are and you can't ask them, that makes things unpleasant. You can always ask some attendings why they are doing something, but you have to read the mood of others. It's all a matter of participation. When you are taken as a colleague, it is very pleasant; but when you are there just to carry out orders and to do the work, then I don't like it (Intern).

Housestaff also feel defenseless against the whims of attendings. They know that there is nothing they can do in the face of an attending's anger. They know that there is nothing they can do when attendings make errors, save talk among themselves. This inequality is, in fact, in one way or another one of their favorite topics of talk. Interestingly enough, it is not the amount of room itself which determines housestaff resentment of attendings. Housestaff can accept very narrow limits if they respect an attending's judgment and skill and if they feel they are learning despite eccentricities that must be tolerated. They then speak of the attending's behavior giving the service "color." On the other hand, housestaff may find relatively more freedom chafing if they do not respect an attending's judgment and if they feel that they are not learning much from a service. This finding parallels Goss's (1961) that professional expertise determines how well or poorly advice is received. Competent professionals need not pull rank since they can persuade by reason.

Now, when you're on Arthur's service, you don't mind too much the way decisions are made. You know Arthur is such a good clinician that even though he's dogmatic, you believe him because he's usually right and when you disagree, you're usually wrong. But with Steele, you argue more because his opinions are not always sound, he makes wrong judgments in the operating room, and his clinical judgment is often poor. Your argue more—it's easier to argue—but since he is less secure, you have less leeway. He's always confused; and when you disagree with him, you feel he is probably wrong (Chief Resident).

On Baker Service, we were having coffee after morning
rounds. Josh was talking about working with different attendings: "It's really funny. When Arthur speaks, it's as if he has
a pipeline from God himself—he's that sure that what he says
is right and the only way to treat a patient; and you don't
think to question him. Then, when you're on Charlie Service,
Henry will tell you with equal conviction an exactly opposite
way of doing things. And when he says it, you believe him"
(Baker Service).

Quasi-normative errors are serious mistakes for subordinates
to make; for them to damage a subordinate, however, he must
make them on more than one service or he must make them
blatantly (see chapter 5 for a fuller discussion). Housestaff are
forgiven an error or two that may reflect a lack of familiarity with
a service. In fact, strong reactions of attendings to these errors is
a way they communicate to housestaff how seriously they take
their personal rules. It is a way of showing what the proper
alignment of roles is, of communicating to housestaff that they
are in the hospital not so much to treat patients as to learn to treat
them. Attendings acknowledge that the system is one in which it
is difficult to be a subordinate:

Surgery is a funny business: You force strong-willed, aggressive, intelligent individuals to become peons. The goal is by
having these individuals sublimate all their own independence,
they will come out five years later as strong individuals with
confidence in their own skills, judgment, and ability
(Attending).

Exogenous Sources
of Failure

Surgical intervention also fails for a number of reasons that do
not implicate the competence of the surgeon in any direct way.
The surgeon's strong sense of individual responsibility has him
turn to these reasons only when the search procedure fails to
reveal any physician error or when the reason is glaringly obvious.
These labels for failure are then a residual category. They raise

no questions of physician competence, deviance, and the social control of performance.

First, there is *failure from disease*. Sometimes the best efforts of surgeons cannot cure those in the more advanced stages of terminal illness. Operative complications always raise questions about the adequacy of surgery; but deaths, especially when separated from the operation by a respectable period of time, do not terribly threaten surgeons. These deaths indicate to surgeons what the limits of their skills are; and they are seen as inevitable. Much disease is irreversible. An interesting feature of the allocation of effort on a surgery ward is the division of patients into two classes: salvageable and nonsalvageable. Heroic care goes only to salvageable patients. The nonsalvageable do not receive emergency cardiac resuscitation or other aggressive life-prolonging measures. This is not to say that the surgeons at Pacific practice euthanasia; rather they limit their heroism. Nonsalvageable patients are allowed to die from their diseases and not saved to suffer from them. These patients are still treated—they are not ignored—but the surgeon does not play all his cards. Salvageable patients are candidates for heroic measures. These two classes of patients help determine the allocation of scarce healing resources.

Second, there is *patient procrastination* or *noncooperation*. Often surgical intervention fails because patients neglect to report symptoms until too late. This happens for a variety of reasons. They may read the symptom correctly and fear the cure —women with breast cancer, for example. They may have religious beliefs that inhibit medical intervention—Christian Scientists, for example. They may not have easy access to health care by virtue of being poor or uninsured. Surgeons view these patients with a mixture of incredulity, compassion, and disgust. Also, patients may report symptoms, consent to care, and then balk at proposed cures—patients facing amputations are an example. These patients refuse to consent to the more radical treatments offered them and agree only to procedures more limited than what the surgeon desires. Here, the surgery performed is a compromise between what the surgeon thinks he can get away with and what the patient will accept as necessary.

On Able Service, Mark and I had left the room of a patient
who had refused to consent to a procedure that White thought
best—a below-the-knee amputation and a dissection of the
lymph nodes in the groin. Despite Mark's best efforts—he
appealed to the patient's responsibility to his family, to his
youthful appearance, and the greater promise for a vigorous
life the more extensive procedure promised, and claimed that
the operation was not as bad as the patient feared—the
patient refused to hear any of it: "You can cut to here and
no further," he said, drawing an imaginary line across his
knee with his hand. When we left the room, I asked Mark if
such refusals were common. He answered: "It happens. It's
rare but it happens. When it happens, I try to explain to the
patient why we want to do the procedure we do. I mean, I
really try to explain so that he understands. I never try to
bullshit somebody into an operation. And then if he still
refuses, I try to work out some compromise that the patient
and I can live with. Now, take this guy: he might be right to
gamble. If I were in his place, I'd accept the knee amputation
and the groin dissection. But I can't say for sure that the
lymph nodes are the source of his problem so I can't in good
conscience play God and demand he have the fuller operation.
He may be right—who knows? As a surgeon, I can't put a gun
to his head and demand that he have what I think is the best
operation" (Able Service).

Here, the patient must share responsibility for the outcome with
the surgeon. The necessity for "informed consent" often com-
promises what the surgeon would like to do.

Third, there is *nursing and support staff error*. Often failure
can be traced to the mistakes of nurses and others involved in
direct patient care. Medication fails to get passed properly; intravenous solutions are not replaced on time, or they are run in too
fast or slow; tests are scheduled but fail to get carried out; blood
samples are contaminated; dressings are not changed promptly
and wounds are not kept clean enough—the list is endless. On the
one hand, subordinates are responsible for seeing that nurses are
mobilized and that work gets done properly; but, on the other
hand, housestaff cannot be responsible for everything everyone

does. So housestaff are held accountable for nursing error that emerges from creating tension with nurses, and they are held accountable for not properly dealing with nursing error. Normal nursing errors are treated by doctors as difficulties in a different chain of command. They are reported to the appropriate authority, and it is assumed that nurses will keep their own house in order.

Fourth, there is *machine malfunction*. Some failures occur because of breakdowns in the enormous technology that supports care in the modern hospital. Computers print out the wrong values for diagnostic tests; ventilators fail; pumps fail. Such things happen, and there is little the surgeon can do, save have the offending machinery replaced or repaired. Failure does not threaten the claim to competence. However, for novices the breakdown of machinery can pose a real threat to confidence. The inexperienced may connect the failure of the machine with a failure of their own skills since they do not have enough practice to form a sense of mastery at the task. The recruit may even feel that the machine is trying to tell him something.

three

Routine Surveillance as Social Control

The typology of error discussed in chapter 2 is an observer's scheme for categorizing how surgeons explain, control, and correct failure. The observer's typification is inadequate in two ways. On the one hand, the typification scheme of surgeons is more subtle. There are many specific varieties of the general type, technical and judgmental errors. There are preoperative, intraoperative, and postoperative techniques and judgments; and each of these is capable of further subdivision so that intraoperatively, for example, surgeons speak of intubating, preparing and draping, opening, clearing the field, making the correction, closing, and extubating as distinct stages of an operation—each with its own set of techniques and judgments and its own calculus of success and failure. On the other hand, the typification scheme of surgeons is more gross. There is only one critical distinction superordinates make in evaluating a failure: was the failure the result of someone doing what any reasonable person in the scene might have done, or was it the result of less than responsible behavior? Error is a dichotomous category. Now, to say that error is both a dichotomous category and a category capable of multiple subdivisions is to say that there is a qualitative difference among errors. Two categories, technical and judgmental, sustain a definition of the situation as normal. Given the necessity for actors to learn by doing, the "surgery is a body-contact sport" philosophy that attendings share with varying degrees of intensity, a mistake assigned to these categories is accepted as routine and inevitable and treated as an occasion for passing on the tricks of the trade. Two categories, normative and quasi-normative, suspend normal definitions of the situation. These are extraordinary errors that challenge the tacit assumptions that make social order possible. A mistake assigned to these categories is treated as a moral breach by a responsible agent and as an occasion for corrective remedies, the most immediately available being the "talking-to" (Freidson and Rhea 1972).

Chapter 2 provides several examples of talking-tos delivered at the time the infraction was discovered. This sanction is so immediately available because it requires an attending physician to mobilize nothing save his outrage. He need not win the approval of his colleagues nor satisfy the requirements of due process nor marshal any evidence beyond what the scene makes immediately available to sustain his claim.

Housestaff report that they find these public talking-tos humiliating; that they make them feel "really worthless"; and that the fear of being a victim motivates performance. At the same time this fear creates bitterness and resentment toward attendings. The mixture of awe and ill will directed at attendings emerges as a common theme in autobiographical accounts of medical training. Especially good examples are found in Cook (1972), Nolen (1970), Glaser (1973), Viscott (1974), and Dr. X (1965).

My cataloging of error in chapter 2 is too taxonomic to give an adequate understanding of the processes by which superiors assign mistakes to one category or another, typify subordinates as responsible or not, and regulate the quality of performance. A taxonomy of mistakes does not reveal the judgmental work done by actors in the scene to construct a reality. In this chapter I hope to remedy that defect. The routine surveillance of action during rounds is the major mode of everyday social control. Rounds are also the least public control as they involve only an attending and his subordinates. Mortality and Morbidity Conferences (see chapter 4) involve an assembly of attendings and subordinates. Promotion decisions (see chapter 5) involve the collegium of attendings. Since rounds serve as the major mode of everyday social controls, it is then that the judgmental work of actors is most apparent. For our purposes three recurring dimensions of rounds behavior are noteworthy: the tension between rule by clinical experience and rule by scientific knowledge; the questioning process; and the place of horror stories in the oral culture of medicine.

Rounds Behavior

There are three different types of rounds that surgeons employ to monitor their performance—work rounds, chart rounds, and attending rounds. Participants in the scene identify at least three other types of rounds. First, there are card rounds, a shortened form of chart rounds. These are a review of a patient's medication. They are often instigated by nurses when prescriptions become outdated and medications are not needed or cannot be dispensed by them legally. As such, card rounds are a nursing control on physician behavior. Second are "chief resident rounds." Alternative terms are used by others, but whatever the designation these are a quick run through the patients with one eye on the clock. Here quickness is the key. (The goal is to reach home before one's children are asleep.) Third are coffee or nutritional rounds. These are held in the cafeteria and usually focus on any and everything, save patients.

Work Rounds

Work rounds are a method for organizing work and allocating effort, as well as checking progress. As a rule, they occur twice daily: like opening and closing exercises in grade school, they are the first and last group projects of the day. On work rounds, subordinates alone participate. In the morning, they decide on what needs to be done that day and they divide the work among themselves. The patients on the service are divided between junior and senior medical students, with interns sharing the load in especially heavy periods. The students have responsibility for completing the most routine work on patients; they are expected to get to know their patients as well as possible in a biomedical sense, but they are also expected to know them well enough as social beings to spot any problems that will interfere with recovery. Medical students are often told by their teachers to get to know patients now because they will never again be in a position to spend so much time with them. To this students reply that it's a shame that the time in their career when they are around the most is the time when they can do the least. All of this routine work is called "scut." The acronym is ironically explained as "some clinically useful training." More complex tasks are reserved for housestaff. Even still, housestaff complain that an inordinate amount of their effort is wasted on tasks beneath their abilities. On afternoon rounds, subordinates regroup, evaluate the results of the day's tests, decide what work is necessary that evening, and reserve the tasks that can wait for the next morning. Also, on afternoon rounds, some extra care is usually made to answer patient questions. The press of a day's work prevents this on morning rounds, which the service rushes through in order to arrive on time at their first appointments.

During work rounds, subordinates are not critical of each other's performance. A joking reproach is the strongest rebuke I ever observed. Housestaff are concerned to make sure that all work is done, that any special requests of the attending have been carried out, and that no troubles have developed that they are unaware of. Improperly done work, missed assignments, and scheduling mix-ups are all seen as group problems. They are everyone's concern and no one's fault. Responsibility for the work of the service is corporate. Nevertheless, this corporate feeling is subject to great strain. There are several factors that predispose attendings to blame junior housestaff for problems. A student is seen as too inexperienced to have major responsibility. A chief resident is too experienced and trustworthy. In addition, attendings have invested five years in a chief resident's training and are committed to believing in his excellence. This leaves interns and second-year residents in the most exposed position, most vulnerable in bad times. In addition, despite the ideal of corporate responsibility, housestaff fear that their colleagues, when confronted by attendings for questionable behavior, will try to shift the blame. They fear being made scapegoats for tasks that fall outside their responsibility:

> There are two ways people make it in academic medicine.
> You can do it on your own ability or by negating the ability of
> others. Too many guys are obsessed with finding a way out.
> You know, saying it's not really my patient or I wasn't on

call last night or something like that. Or they'll go back and find an abnormal lab value in some old test and then argue that it [the death or complication] was happening all along and their decisions were not what did it (Intern).

Josh and the rest of the Baker Service gathered in the conference room after being dressed down by Arthur for shoddy performance. Arthur claimed that the kindest thing that could be said about their work was that it was "disinterested" and the strongest that it "borders on criminal malpractice." All of the service felt that nothing they had done justified such an outburst. They all commented on this. One of the junior students regretted that Ernest, the chief resident, had missed rounds because he would have known how to handle Arthur; the student expressed the hope that when Arthur spoke with Ernest, the chief resident would be able to explain things and straighten things out. Josh Carter, the resident second-in-command, answered, "Fat chance! Don't bet on it. No, Ernest will tell Arthur that he's been letting me run the service. Yeah, I bet that's what he tells him. You'll see, I'm the one who's going to wind up getting screwed" (Baker Service).

Despite this fear of being made a scapegoat, it is rare in actual practice. In fact, as the text below makes clear, a very real opposite danger exists that problems cannot be shifted to those to whom they rightfully belong. One reason is that attendings do not accept such accounts as legitimate:

Forget the resident who says, "I don't know what happened—it was my night off." He'll never make it. I say that in the army there were only three answers you could give: "Yes, sir"; "No, sir"; and "No excuse, sir." That's true for surgery, too (Attending).

For attendings, the way that subordinates divide work is immaterial; quality performance is demanded; and lapses are everyone's responsibility. Because of this, attendings do not believe that housestaff can be asked unfair questions about actions taken on the service. A response that denies responsibility or knowledge is unacceptable for it communicates to attendings a disinterest in clinical care.

Work rounds are then a method that subordinates employ to protect themselves as a corporate group. This activity guarantees that each member of the service will see each patient daily, regardless of his individual responsibility for the patient.

The information exchanged during rounds is a capsule summary of the salient facts of a patient's clinical history. The informal division of labor has members of the service take turns assuming primary responsibility for patients admitted to the service. This random method of matching patient and subordinate is seen as the most equitable way of distributing both "scut work" and interesting cases. The rule of assignment, "Your turn—your patient," is interpreted in much the same way as the rule of assignment in a welfare office that Zimmerman (1970) discusses, both in its application and in its breach. If a service member feels he has an oversupply of cases that are purely scut, he may request a patient whom he feels is interesting; or if a service member feels an embarrassment of riches with regard to interesting cases, he may volunteer for a patient ill with an uninteresting disease. The member of the service with responsibility for the patient according to the informal division of labor among subordinates recites the following: when the patient is new and has not yet been introduced to the service, the patient's initial complaint and proposed plan of treatment; and, once the service knows a patient, his medications and their indications; the latest lab reports, with a special emphasis on important or abnormal lab values, the plan and schedule of treatment for the patient, and any other relevant and unusual information about the patient, such as dietary restrictions or secondary problems.

Basically, work rounds circulate the information that everyone who treats the patient should know to the entire group of subordinates. Work rounds provide a patient with ongoing treatment and they allow housestaff to be in command of the situation. They rehearse leadership and decision making. They also rehearse attending rounds which are, as we shall see, a competence test. In surgical training, in all clinical education, the patient is the subject matter which must be mastered. Work rounds are a group review session. Medical education is in some sense a paradigm of an open classroom, at least in its clinical aspects. On the service first- through seventh-year students are working at tasks, mastering them, and then moving on to tasks of greater complexity. Further, it is often the individual who has recently learned who passes on his newfound knowledge. This idyll of self-learning suffers some tensions. Some individuals feel they progress too slowly. Sometimes discussion passes over the heads of the least experienced; other times it cannot sustain the interest of the most experienced. Always, there is the problem of overload. The peer network that evolves is not unlike the one that Bossert (1975) describes for third- and fourth-graders in open classrooms.

Chart Rounds

In addition to work rounds, housestaff prepare themselves for attending rounds and monitor their own work by chart rounds. Here, housestaff review a patient's medical records. Chart rounds serve a number of purposes. First, they allow housestaff to trace the natural history of disease processes. Second, they provide a quick and efficient way of keeping up to date on a patient's condition without ever seeing the patient. From the chart, the housestaff member can often glean all the information about patients necessary for his purposes at hand. In fact, housestaff comment that really good charting and nursing makes their actually seeing patients unnecessary.

> Ernest and I were heading for the Intensive Care Unit to see Mr. Grotesk, a patient who had had a cardiac arrest the night before. As we were talking down the corridor Ernest said to me: "The thing about the ICU is that when you get a really good nurse, you never have to see the patient. You can ask a few questions about blood gases, vital signs, and urine output, read the chart, and look at a few numbers and you'll know everything you need to know" (Baker Service).

Third, in cases where little progress has been made, service members use chart rounds to search for new clues to an illness that they have not yet understood. Fourth, and most important, chart rounds are a way housestaff have of checking the thoroughness, skill, understanding, and reliability of the medical students on the service. The major part of the student's responsibility consists of charting the findings from the patient's physical examination. The student's clinical impressions are written up and added to the patient's record. For the student, this is practice in diagnosis. The student's results are then checked by a member of the housestaff, who repeats the examination of the patient for himself. Housestaff use chart rounds to monitor the performance of students. Part of the review is of the actual clinical findings and part of it is of the art of chart writing. Since so much medical communication is in this medium, the second part of this review is not unimportant. Charts provide a running record of subordinate performance. However, we never observed attendings indexing poor performance by a retrospective reading of charts. Nevertheless, as Freidson and Rhea (1972) point out, the clinical record is always latently supervisory.

Attending Rounds

Attending rounds occur at the pleasure of the attending: on the Able Service, this was once a week; on the Baker Service, it was three or five days a week. The attendings of the other two surgical services made more rounds than the attendings of Able but less than those of Baker. These rounds are the occasion when patients are visited by attendings, when the lessons of clinical experience are passed on, when a pretense of discussion before decision making is provided, and when attendings match their own clinical impressions against those of their housestaff and, in cases of discrepancy, seek accounts. Made to do different work for different people—they provide reassurance and comfort for patients, teaching for students, colleagueship for housestaff, and a stage for attending performances—these rounds have a strong social control component. Attending rounds are, if nothing else, a poking around on the part of superordinates to make certain that their houses are kept in order. When the service is running smoothly, the teaching, collegial, and humane work of rounds can be accomplished. That is to say, these tasks are attended to only when social control is unnecessary or completed. The social

control component of rounds is usually routinely disposed of.
I did notice in those cases where this was not so that attendings
did not lessen patient contact; if anything, they expanded it. Perhaps they felt that if their housestaff were not doing things right,
then *they* would have to do everything. Because clinical dialogue
is so embedded in the environment, the testlike quality of rounds
is sometimes lost on participants. The way social control is built
into rounds allows for less threatening definitions of reality than
competence testing.

Attending rounds are governed by a formal etiquette that gives
their enactment a ceremonial flavor. First, the members of the
service file into the patient's room in order of rank: attendings
followed by housestaff in order of years of experience followed by
students. The exit pattern is the same. The only variation in this
ritualized coming and going is minor and is a function of the very
human problem of fitting so much human traffic through such a
narrow space as a doorway.[1] At any rate, this traffic pattern never
varies with regard to attendings. They are always the first in and
the first out. Next, if an attending has never met a patient before,
the houseofficer who is responsible for the patient introduces him
in a stylized fashion:

> "Dr. X, meet Mr. Morris. Mr. Morris is a fifty-two-year-old
> male who was admitted with a possible gastric ulcer. His vital
> signs are good. His chemistries are not yet back from the
> lab. We have scheduled a small bowel series for tomorrow
> and a large bowel series the day after that."

The attending then shakes hands with the patient, asks him a few
questions, makes a quick physical exam, and assures the patient
he can help him. Attendings state that this laying on of hands is
as much for the patient's benefit—to satisfy his expectation of
what doctors do—as for anything the doctors hope to learn.
Moreover, cheerful assurance is only one of a number of possible
interaction styles. It is the one attendings of both the Able and
Baker Service preferred. An alternative style that has been discussed is "hanging crepe" (Siegler 1975). When an attending
hangs crepe, he paints a hopeless case and offers only mild hope

that he can salvage the situation. There is, I think, reason to believe that there is a positive bias in surgeons' interaction styles. Partly this is a denial of the possibility of failure. Partly this is a device to mobilize the patient's healing resources and cooperation. The surgeon who told his patient, "Good God, I don't think you're going to make it. I just hope you don't die on the table" would win neither friends nor awards for his bedside manner. The importance of individual action predisposes surgeons to aggressive confidence more than other physicians who are not so personally committed to their interventions and who are more tolerant of the natural course of disease. If an attending has met a patient, he asks him a few questions and then turns to his subordinates. He asks the group questions about patient care and about recent literature bearing on the patient's condition. The person who has responsibility for the patient is expected by the group to field these questions. Occasionally, attendings will direct questions to particular individuals, especially when their performance is suspect.

If all questions put to housestaff are answered satisfactorily and if things appear in order, then knowledge of good performance builds. Housestaff become trusted. In the future, more time on rounds is spent teaching and being collegial with subordinates. If things appear awry and housestaff cannot explain why, attendings spend greater time on the social control of performance. Housestaff are not trusted. The distrust of subordinates is a consequence of the way they acquit themselves on rounds:

> You look at the way patients are approached. You try to find out if your housestaff know what's going on. Say Mrs. X has been a patient for three days and you ask about Mrs. X's chest X ray and they haven't seen it. Then you feel that they don't know what's going on. Or say Mrs. X has been in a lot of pain and they don't know about it. You don't expect your young people to know all the answers to all the problems; but you expect them to know what the problems are. You expect them to know what is happening and why. When you find they don't, you begin to check things more closely. You look

at the dressings to see if they are bothering themselves with keeping them clean (Attending).

Stelling and Bucher (1972) have defined the zone of autonomy that surrounds subordinates as "elastic"; that is to say, monitoring and performance covary. Quite clearly, monitoring is related to the evaluation of performance; indeed, monitoring itself may be a deviance-amplifying mechanism (see Wender 1968). It is deviance-amplifying because when an attending feels the need to increase monitoring he is already convinced that something is wrong. What is wrong are the signs that housestaff are not getting the job done. Attendings notice, for example, that wounds are not dressed properly; that scheduling problems are developing and that tests are not being done; that lungs are not cleared vigorously enough following surgery; or that women are not made to exercise their arms following mastectomies. The attending then surveys patients more intensively and questions housestaff more closely and more often about the actual quantity of their effort as opposed to the theoretic quality of that effort. In such cases, the attending is more likely to find errors. Those that he finds he is more likely to brand as normative or quasi-normative. He finds them because he is looking for them and because he is sure they are there for the finding. On the other hand, when the attending feels that the service is in order, the questions he raises are limited and confined to the theoretic justification for action. In this case an attending finds technical and judgmental errors; he finds these because at least for the moment his housestaff are above suspicion of more serious breaches.

A consequence of this pattern of surveillance is that during periods of high monitoring, housestaff often feel that they are being unfairly treated by attendings. Their resentment of their subordinate and defenseless position grows, and they begin to form assessments of attendings as capricious, arbitrary individuals who are impossible to please or understand:

The members of the Baker Service were complaining about their most recent dressing-down by Dr. Arthur. Josh Carter was visibly upset; he sat apart from the group and chain-smoked. Darwin, the senior student, offered him support: "Look. You know with Arthur it takes only one thing to go wrong for him to jump up and down all over you. And once he finds something, he nit-picks until he finds a whole raft of things. Maybe if Jerome's wound hadn't been shut and with paper tape at that, then maybe we would have made it." (Using paper tape on the Baker Service is a quasi-normative error.) This prompted the junior student who had mistakenly taped the wound shut to apologize to Carter. Carter replied, "It's okay, really it is. If the wound hadn't been taped shut, then he would have found something else. Really, it's not your fault. If it hadn't been this, it would have been something else. That son-of-a-bitch is just a malevolent bastard" (Baker Service).

The housestaff perception that the attending was just looking for something to complain about is correct but it is also incomplete. Housestaff neglect to explain why the attending would be motivated to look for something to begin with. For their part, attendings look for problems because, following their rule of "forgive and remember," they discern a pattern in the work around them and failures can no longer be considered random clinical events. So the fact that without advance warning attendings step up monitoring, become more dogmatic about the way they want work done, and more critical of subordinates is not arbitrary. It may appear so to the subordinate who is not aware that an attending has changed his interpretation of a subordinate's performance from favorable to unfavorable and reread past events in this light. The subordinate is after all doing what he has done all along and this has always been acceptable in the past.

Moreover, there is a predictable temporal patterning to the surveillance of performance on a rotation. At first, monitoring is rather complete as the attending lays down the law in the beginning. He defines his expectations for subordinate performance. Then, the attending withdraws somewhat. If things go well, surveillance relaxes and at the end of a rotation, housestaff-attending relations are relaxed and cordial. However, if things go poorly, then the attending steps in again and provides tighter control. In such cases at the end of a rotation, relations among housestaff and attendings are strained, highly formal, and very unequal:

> When you have problems with an attending, they will declare themselves at the end of a rotation and they are really a matter of no longer communicating with an attending. Of course, attendings bawl you out, humiliate you—that's part of training. Some, however, go beyond that. They order too many tests; they make too much work; they show poor judgment in the operating room. When that happens, it's best to stay away from them as much as possible (Chief Resident).

But it is precisely at this point that the attending is most difficult to avoid because this is when he is paying the most attention to work. He may not appear any more often—Dr. Peters never makes rounds more than once a week—however, the time spent is more intense; the attending spends more time asking questions about each patient and he spends more time getting clinical readings of his own. As a consequence, the attending has more direct orders to give. Furthermore, to the extent that the attending takes charge of a patient's care, a subordinate has his autonomy usurped.

Clinical Experience vs. Scientific Reasoning

It is through a system of such give-and-take that attendings evaluate housestaff, regulate performance, and identify deviant housestaff—those who cannot meet the demands of a surgical career. The power of the attending is most noteworthy. On the basis of his observations on rounds, however hastily they might be made, the superordinate encroaches on the autonomy of subordinates by countermanding orders and reproving behavior. In the process, careers are made and broken. This almost total control of action in the scene is a power and privilege of rank. As judgmental and quasi-normative errors indicate, the word of the attending is law. The attending may not always be right; but in cases where he finds himself disagreeing with his housestaff, he need not give good reasons for his preferences. To have them acted out, he need only announce them. On the other hand, the good reasons of a subordinate are in themselves never a sufficient cause for attendings to embark on a course of action. This is to say, that in disputes over what a clinical reality is, the attending has the last word. He has the right to construct reality as he sees fit. The subordinate is compelled for all practical purposes to accept this definition of reality, however much he may resent it, distrust it, or disagree with it. This power of the attending to construct the binding interpretation of reality has powerful control implications. It means that the attending whose professional behavior is improper is beyond the reach of any subordinate who notices it. Subordinates' notions of the justice of a system of professional control rests on the faith that such behavior cannot long remain secret and in time other attendings will know of and be forced to act on this guilty knowledge. At the same time, houseofficers themselves are defenseless against whatever charges an attending may level. The completion of their own training rests on the hope that attendings will be tolerant and forgiving of their errors. In this situation the power of an attending and its restraint are striking. In rounds behavior, we are able to see what beliefs legitimate this power, what beliefs restrain it, and what tensions underlie it. There are two competing systems of legitimation for medical authority: clinical expertise and scientific evidence.[2] These systems are not of equal importance: in the case of discrepant opinions, arguments based on clinical expertise override those based on scientific evidence.[3] Such a system of legitimation concentrates power in the person of the attending. On the one hand, he is the active creator of the most recent scientific evidence; in some specific cases the attending is literally the last word on a subject. On the other hand, by virtue of his clinical experience, he knows when scientific findings are not appropriate for charting a course of action. He knows the rules and their exceptions. The subordinate is learning the rules; he does not yet have enough experience to recognize the exceptions.

Rule by scientific evidence alone implies a more egalitarian and formally rational legitimation of authority; and as a consequence, a more formally rational task-structure. Ironically, this mode of legitimation alone is both less collegial and more egalitarian. In such a system, all arguments have equal weight; the authority of evidence and the authority of the person who presents it are independent. Subordinates who read widely are in a position to challenge an attending's authority and increase their own autonomy. Thus, those in the training situation would have more equal access to the source of legitimate authority. However, because of the greater importance of clinical expertise, superordinates are in a position to reject scientific evidence that they feel violates their own sense of what the situation requires:

> We were visiting Mr. Darnell, who had a proctocolectomy [removal of rectum and distal end of colon with externalization of proximal colon] the day before. As Arthur was surveying the wound, Ernest asked him about a new technique developed by Dr. Stanley and reported in a recent journal article. According to Ernest, Stanley reported that on a series of patients using this new technique, he had no instances of a particular complication. Arthur replied: "I've tried that technique and I've seen patients on whom it was used, and I'm convinced it's not a bit better." Ernest repeated: "But in a large series, there were no complications." Arthur answered: "Then Stanley has a poor memory, or he didn't include in his series at least six of his patients I treated for that complication." Ernest asked: "Doesn't that call for a letter to the editor, sir?" Arthur answered: "I don't think it would do much good. Dr. Stanley is the editor" (Baker Service).

The point of the above vignette is not that medical researchers falsify their results and, unless one is careful, one will be misled.[4] More likely, Arthur was having some fun at Stanley's expense (Stanley was a former attending at Pacific). He was using humor to pass a lesson on to his subordinates: the logic of your own experience determines the usefulness of the research of others.

Scientific evidence takes its meaning in the light of the current
clinical situation and past clinical experience.

The passing on of clinical expertise also allows for a more
collegial relation to develop than scientific evidence alone provides. It allows superordinates to induct subordinates into the
secrets of the profession. Often attendings on rounds will ask
subordinates to project a clinical plan of action, praise them for
the formal correctness of their answers, and then point out how
such plans are nevertheless inappropriate given the nature of the
situation:

> Mrs. Sharper was admitted complaining of abdominal pain.
> She had been operated on twice at another hospital in the
> area and to Arthur it was "obvious" that her problems were
> iatrogenic. He claimed that of the two surgeons who had
> operated on her earlier, the first is a "heavy-handed son-of-a-
> bitch," and the second is "untalented, but he married
> well." Then Arthur asked Christian what he thought should
> be done. Christian replied that he would like to run a series
> of tests to determine the extent of the damage and that then
> they should go in and make the necessary correction, revising
> the work of the other surgeons.
>
> Arthur replied that under ideal conditions, Christian was
> right; but for this patient it would be unwise to revise the
> damage of the earlier surgeons. They should go in and relieve
> her difficulty and they should do that stat [immediately].
> Arthur said that this should be done not because it was a life-
> threatening situation nor because it was an emergency, but
> because "Mrs. Sharper is a seventy-four-year-old woman and
> when you get old people in the hospital, put them on their
> backs in bed, start running IV tubes into them, and plac-
> ing nasogastric tubes down them, they die. It never fails. The
> best thing to do with old people is to get them in and out of
> the hospital as quickly as possible."
>
> To give evidence for this assertion, Arthur told the story of
> an experience that he had as an intern, one that had made "a
> damn strong impression on him, one that he'd never forget."
> The story went as follows: One of his first rotations was on

the service of a surgeon who did prostate operations for
wealthy patients at "a thousand a shot." Arthur claimed,
"Now, that's a lot of money but well worth it if your bladder
is obstructed." One of Arthur's first patients was an old man
needing a prostate operation done, but he also had com-
plicating problems that required extensive tests. And, as
Arthur related it, "That son-of-a-bitch died before we had a
chance to operate." Arthur learned the following lesson from
the experience which he passed on to the group: "While I
am as you know quite conservative about preoperative care
[*conservative* here means he requires a lot], for old people,
like this lady, just get them in and out as fast as possible before they die on you. Fart around and they'll die. I swear it.
It never fails" (Baker Service).

Mrs. Hooper, a patient on the Able Service, has a huge lump
in the groin area. Dr. White asked Paul what course of action
he would recommend if the lump turned out to be a sarcoma
[a malignant tumor of the muscle]. Paul answered that he
thought hip disarticulation [removal of leg at hip joint]
would be the operation of choice. White agreed that it would
be the operation of choice, but stated that he would not
recommend it in this case: "I don't think this lady could live
with a hip disarticulation. She's relatively obese and I don't
think that she would tolerate the procedure very well. She'd
be confined to a wheelchair the rest of her life. I've had
patients do remarkably well with hip disarticulation, but not
in this case. I think I'll just have to scoop it out as best I
can." He then added facetiously, "Maybe it's cat-scratch
fever. There's a big run on cat scratches these days."
"Unfortunately she doesn't have a cat," said Paul. "I know,"
answered White. "But I think we can get good results
scooping it out. I once had a patient with an invasive tumor
that I just kept scooping out. I was able to save his leg for ten
years that way," added Dr. Peters (Able Service).

Through such exchanges, attendings communicate to subordinates a number of messages. First, they pass on what considerations should lead one to modify conventional wisdom. Second,
they allow attendings to support a subordinate's performance
on one level while, on another level, they allow the attending to

change it. The attending's citation of lessons learned from his own clinical history indicates to subordinates how much they have left to learn. Third, these exchanges communicate a certain, albeit limited, sympathy that attendings have for the plight of their subordinates. In such exchanges one of the things that a superordinate is telling his subordinate is, "Look, we all learn the hard way. I did; you will."

> On Able Service, we entered Mrs. Grout's room, a patient with metastatic cancer. While in the hospital she was given penicillin for a secondary infection. Although she reported no known history of allergy and although there was nothing in the official record to indicate an allergy, she had an allergic reaction—hives, swollen face, and cold sores. Dr. Peters looked at her, told her she was doing much better, and left her room. Outside he said to Mark, "Sure is something, isn't it? Well, there's no way you could have known. I remember the first time I had a patient have an allergic reaction. Really made me respect the stuff. Made me very cautious about using it. I daresay that you'll think twice in the future before prescribing it." Mark said he would (Able Service).

This last message that the invocation of clinical expertise carried with it is rarely so forcefully stated as above. As a consequence, it is subject to much noise and distortion. Subordinates are often more aware of the critical rather than the supportive import of being overruled. Housestaff complain that they are not allowed to participate fully enough in decision making and that when an attending's actions are not supported by the facts, there is nothing they can do. In addition, the fact that arguments from personal clinical experience are compelling means that the attending is drawing on a store of private knowledge not available to subordinates. This reinforces in the mind of housestaff the stereotype of the arbitrary attending.

For their part, subordinates rely on scientific evidence to ground their decisions. This is quite natural since their stock of firsthand knowledge is so small. Sudnow (1967) notes the importance of "counting" in a hospital. Any individual counts events, that is, sees them as unique occurrences whose characteristics need attending to, until events of this type become for him a routine taken-for-granted part of the environment. In Sudnow's study, a veteran hospital worker is the one who has lost count of the deaths he has seen; a novice still counts and still catalogs—he still notices death. If Icheiser (1972) did not remind us that we are never so blind as when we are facing the "obvious," it might strike us as strange that persons die and others not notice. But a good working definition of a hospital is that place where death occurs and no one notices; or, more sharply, the place where others agree to notice death as a social fact only so far as it fits their particular purposes.

On a service there is great variation in the degree to which one notices death. Attendings and chief residents have stopped counting deaths; in all likelihood, junior medical students are so clinically uninitiated that they have not yet seen anyone die first-hand—they are ready to begin counting.

As far as it fits their particular purposes, for surgeons death ends their action. It is not unfair to recognize that there is a gladiator dimension to surgery and surgeons. Surgeons take up scalpel against disease; they resist with force its invasion on the body. When death comes, the struggle is ended. Little is said to the patient's family. Like prideful Achilles, the surgeon repairs to his tent and prepares for his next combat. Surgeons are not unaware of this dimension of their work. When one asks a surgeon why he chose to do this of all things medical, invariably in his reply he mentions the dramatic and decisive interventions that are the surgeon's. Surgeons report that they like being "where the action is" (Goffman 1961).

I mention this only to point out a relationship between task-structure and the moral and ethical division of labor. By and large, surgeons have not been contributors to the literature on death and dying. This is not by accident nor does it discredit the surgeon. Surgeons live within the bounds of a simple code; they view it as the task of others to articulate philosophies.

Exposure to clinical problems are the events that are significant enough for housestaff to keep track of, to count: a porta-

caval shunt [a connection of the main vein from the intestine to
the main vein from the lower body bypassing the liver], a hemi-
pelvectomy [removal of lower extremity and half the pelvis], for a
malignant schwannoma [a tumor of the nerve], a case of Zollin-
ger-Ellison syndrome [a tumor of the pancreas which causes the
stomach to secrete excess acid], or a gastroenterostomy [a connection of stomach to upper intestine], are big events in a houseofficer's development. Each new event provides impressions to
match against the clinical descriptions in the literature and each
exposure provides knowledge that can be used next time. Housestaff proceed by the book because they have not yet developed an
overly large and useful stock of knowledge. Yet following procedures—going by the book—has a virtue all its own: as long as
one has done this, one is protected from the damaging interpretations of failure. Better to blame bad luck than *hubris*:

> Mark had performed an esophagogastrectomy [removal of
> esophagus and stomach], on Mr. Warren. This was Mark's
> first, and he was being generally left alone by Arthur and
> Grant to manage the patient. (Mark's training has only six
> weeks left and the attendings are treating him very much as
> a colleague.) Mark has a special interest in Mr. Warren. His
> chief concern was whether his anastomosis would hold. He
> had taped a note to Mr. Warren's forehead forbidding any-
> one from moving the tube placed down Warren's nose, his
> fear being that the tube would rip the suture line. We were
> visiting Mr. Warren on morning rounds. Mark was pleased
> to see that there were no difficulties in the immediate post-
> operative period. Stan asked him when he intended to feed
> Mr. Warren. "Seven days," Mark answered. "You know
> Gray [an attending noted for his skill at this procedure] has
> them eating much faster than that. On the third day postop
> he already has them on clear liquids," Stan said. "I know,
> but let me try that and have it not work. They'd crucify me.
> Unh, unh! I want no part of that. Because, after all, this is
> only my hundred and first [with a heavy emphasis on *first*]
> esophagogastrectomy. I'm going to play it really straight"
> (Baker Service).

The guidelines in the scientific literature establish a standard of proper behavior for housestaff. The attending who does not follow these standards and cannot supply acceptable reasons for his deviations is often viewed by housestaff as "dogmatic" or "lacking in clinical judgment." The attending who does not follow these standards but can give acceptable reasons, that is, can extract generalizable lessons from his clinical experience, is respected by housestaff as a good teacher. Much more autocratic and much more eccentric behavior is tolerated without complaint in the second case than in the first.

The tension between clinical expertise and scientific evidence expresses the inequalities among ranks on a surgery service; it also expresses an even more basic tension of medical practice: the art of healing versus the science of medicine. Rule by clinical expertise emphasizes the "artful" dimensions of practice. The attending's claim of authority has an almost mystical quality: "Trust me, for I have seen." In the world of medicine, clinical acumen is a charismatic possession, a gift of grace; its exact nature is a mystery. On the other hand, rule by scientific evidence emphasizes the rational and technical dimensions of practice. The legitimation of scientific evidence is of the most routine nature; the exact nature of this authority is not mysterious but known to all. Operationally, these two types of legitimation are resources that actors in a scene possess to justify a course of action. Attendings possess both types of authority. In contrast, their subordinates have little science, less clinical expertise. As a consequence, attendings always have the unanswerable argument. Although an attending's authority is in some formal sense always legitimate, unless his authority is respected by virtue of both his clinical and scientific expertise, then his subordinates are likely to experience his leadership as interference, to avoid his control whenever possible, and to grouse to others about the attending's shortcomings.

Subordinates resent the attending's power to construct a binding definition of reality for good reason. One of those binding definitions that an attending makes is whether or not an individual should be allowed to progress through training. At-

tending rounds are an occasion for the attending to determine
through questioning the sophistication of a subordinate's reasoning, to observe whether a subordinate works hard enough to get
adequate results, to appraise if a subordinate has any personality
problems that prevent him from doing decent work, and to
judge in general whether the subordinate promises to be worth
the effort it takes to train a surgeon. This judgment is legitimated
on the basis of the clinical expertise an attending has developed
through his teaching experience. As with the invocation of clinical expertise in patient care, the subordinate has no remedies if
he finds himself in disagreement with clinical wisdom. If he is
asked to leave a training program, the subordinate cannot appeal
the decision, show how it was biased and the facts of the situation
misread, and then be reinstated. The dismissed subordinate
must find a place somewhere else or give up any hope of becoming a board-certified surgeon.[5] The fact that such decisions
are legitimated by clinical expertise means that they are both
unanswerable and unanalyzable—they are as mysterious as the
source of this authority. Not surprisingly, this is a major resentment and tension of housestaff before they enter the upper end of
the pyramid and are relatively secure:

> I really dislike the autocratic nature of surgery. Attendings
> piss you off and there's nothing you can do. And if you piss
> attendings off they can screw you. Some attendings are really
> vindictive. They have no concern for us at all (Resident).

> On Baker Service, Arthur had complained bitterly after
> rounds about the quality of work. Josh had felt the criticism
> was unfair and he complained to me: "Let me tell you some-
> thing: this is a pyramid program and in a few weeks these
> guys are going to sit down and decide who to keep for senior
> residents. And when you get kicked out of a program you
> don't move to Mass. General. You move laterally if you're
> lucky, really lucky, or you move downward. You make one
> public enemy like this bastard and he can ruin your career. I
> don't know what it's like for you in graduate school, but if
> you want to get through this training program you'd better be
> prepared to swallow a whole lot of shit." I assured him there

was some shit in graduate school and asked if there was any way to disagree with an attending. "How can you? It doesn't matter if you're right; they can still screw you. The only time you could do anything is if you decided that you didn't want to stay here and you really didn't care where you went next. Then maybe you could hit back when they lash out at you. But as it is now you have no choice but to take whatever they dish out without being able to defend yourself. It doesn't matter whether you're right or wrong or anything. You just have to take it (Baker Service).

The fact that clinical judgment is the basis for evaluation unsettles housestaff. They see decisions concerning patient management that seem arbitrary and contrary to the demands of science justified by clinical expertise; they are dressed-down for quasi-normative errors which are mistakes only from the idiosyncratic perspective of an individual attending; and they see that their interpretation of events is of little importance. Because of this, they fear the possibility of being unfairly evaluated; and because these evaluations are on such relatively unspecified grounds, those dismissed may always claim they were unfairly treated, the victims of a malevolent attending. The intensity of these beliefs may blind us to another function of clinical expertise—that is, such expertise is also the basis of the toleration and forgiveness of subordinate errors. The attending's judgment in these cases does not alienate his subordinates but rather creates strong allegiances and debts that subordinates must repay by a higher standard of work in the future. What we are concerned with at present is, given such a system of authority, how does the attending construct a judgment of his subordinates? How do ward rounds function as a competence quiz? This brings us to the questioning process by which superordinates test subordinates.

The Questioning Process

To understand how attendings judge the performance of subordinates, it is necessary to examine how subordinates are questioned. To do so, we have to recall two considerations developed

above: (1) there are two different orders of failure: an account
either sustains or subverts a normal definition of the situation;
and (2) an attending by virtue of the preeminence of clinical
expertise has the right to construct the binding interpretation of
reality—an attending need not modify his claims about what is
happening because of the counterclaims of housestaff. Given
this, we may speak of how meanings about the quality of performance are negotiated, all the time recognizing that there are
limits to the meaningfulness of calling these negotiations since an
attending can break off discussion at any point.

Basically, we can describe the questioning process on rounds as
an attempt to establish to what order subordinate performance
belongs: is a subordinate failing to meet minimal role requirements and by such behavior making normative or quasi-normative breaches; or is he a reasonable and responsible subordinate
whose only errors are the technical and judgmental errors of
inexperience? The chief weapon that the attending uses to find
out is the question. As Sacks's chain-rule for questions establishes
(Churchill 1971), the proper etiquette for question-answer-ques-
tion-answer sequences is, after the reply, the floor belongs to the
questioner. Linguistic practice here subserves the needs of social
rank. The superordinate can and does question subordinates until
he receives an account that renders further questions unnecessary
for his purposes. In a sense then, the attending's control of
resources is extraordinary—not only can he construct a binding
definition of reality, but there are no inherent limits which he
must respect in questioning his subordinates.

Earlier I stated that the amount of monitoring is inversely
related to an attending's evaluation of a subordinate. We must
now go beyond this generalization and see how the judgment that
performance is either acceptable or not is constructed on a
day-to-day basis on rounds. When work is proceeding without incident and after subordinates have earned the trust of superordinates, there is not much monitoring of performance. There is a
relaxed tone to decision making. Subordinates find it easier to
tolerate the whims of superordinates, and superordinates find the
gestures for independence of subordinates more acceptable:

On morning work rounds, we were in Mrs. Morrow's room. Mark ordered that her subclavian line [an intravenous tube from arm into large veins in neck] be discontinued. "I don't think you want to do that, Mark," John said. "Why?" John: "Yesterday on rounds, Grant [Mrs. Morrow's attending] said he wanted it kept until she's eating a lot." Mark: "Okay. Keep it in. I can't see what difference it makes either way." As we left the room, Stan began talking to me. "I guess you've noticed that when things are going well, our decisions are not terribly important. Whether an IV is in for a day or so longer, whether a patient is on clear or full liquids, it doesn't matter much so long as they are getting better. But when things are bad, and life is at stake, then these same decisions are crucial" (Baker Service).

Surgeons do not like to disturb success any more than anyone else. When there is little at stake for participants, routine and minor encroachments of autonomy are easily tolerated. In fact, as long as things go on smoothly, such little things tend to go unnoticed by actors.

However, when work is not proceeding smoothly or when it is early in a rotation and subordinates have not yet earned the trust of attendings, rounds can be a very intense competence quiz with a complete accounting for action demanded. After attendings have sniffed around some by inspecting dressings and wounds and by listening to lung fields and the like, questioning begins. First, are questions of a general nature, such as "How is this patient doing?" Equally general answers, such as "Fine," do not suffice:

I'm sure you've heard me ask, "How's this patient?" and heard someone answer "Fine." Well, I don't want impressions. I want the facts. If someone says a patient is fine— especially if I don't trust them—I'll ask further: "What are the blood counts?" Anyone can say a patient is fine, but that doesn't tell you much about your patient (Attending).

Look—you've heard us say on rounds, "Don't give me impressions. I don't give a good goddamn how a patient looks. Give me numbers" (Attending).

The subordinate who answers superordinate questions with vague responses is presumed to be covering his ignorance, while the subordinate who answers general questions with technically complete responses or who, in informing an attending of a change in a patient's condition, is as complete as possible wins an attending's trust:

> The intern who calls you up and says X has a fever does not inspire your trust; but the intern who calls and says X has a urinary tract infection is altogether different. He reports the symptoms, gives you his diagnosis, and tells you what he plans to do. I don't need housestaff to tell me my patients have fevers—any secretary can do that—good housestaff take a little more initiative (Attending).

The subordinate who requires further questioning has by this fact alone led an attending to question his competence and trustworthiness. The attending must spend a great effort on this subordinate just to get an accurate reading of the situation. Questions follow in rapid succession: What are the blood counts? What did the latest chest film show? When is the barium swallow scheduled? Such questions are an attempt to establish if a subordinate at least knows what is going on with a patient. If a subordinate knows the facts of a case, questioning can move on to questions of treatment; but if a subordinate does not know what is going on with a patient, then the reason for this must be established. Here, there is only one acceptable defense: "The lab has not completed the test yet." Any other excuse such as "It's not my patient" or "I was off last night" indicate to an attending that a subordinate is not putting forth minimal effort to meet the requirements of his role. When such excuses are offered, an attending often dresses-down his subordinate. When the subordinate offers no excuses, the subordinate may be spared the dressing-down, although the attending usually finds other indirect methods for communicating his displeasure. Common tactics are to ignore the offender—literally to act as if he were not there—or to be exaggeratedly formal. In either case, the superordinate steps up monitoring. This results in an attending finding more and more things not to his liking. It is this that is the deviance-amplifying effect of monitoring: the actual rate of unacceptable practice may not increase, but the number of discovered instances rises. A very similar thing may be going on in the current malpractice crisis. It seems very unlikely that the rise in suits reflects an actual rise in negligent practice. More likely, a heightened sensitivity on the part of the lay public to the possibility that bad results are the consequence of bad practice encourages the suit as a remedy. What the rise in suits may speak to is a weakening of the physician's charisma and the evolution of a more formally contractual physician-patient relationship. There is a second striking parallel to this stepped-up monitoring of physicians: complaints about fee-seeking attorneys are similar to those housestaff make of attendings.

Once a subordinate establishes that he knows the facts of a case, questioning moves on to the next level, treatment. Here the subordinate must demonstrate that he knows what medications the patient is receiving and for what indications. A subordinate's ignorance is again evidence for an attending that the subordinate is not meeting the minimal requirements of his role. From this, it is not a great distance that an attending must travel logically to conclude that errors do not result from inexperience but from lack of concern for the norms and quasi-norms of good clinical practice. The subordinate who is found wanting here is in trouble in at least the short run and perhaps the long. Subordinates for their part feel that there are good reasons to explain why they might not know what is going on in any particular patient. They are angered by the attending's refusal to give these accounts a hearing. They complain that attendings are insensitive to physical demands placed on them:

> Carl was upset about Thelma Halsted's death. He blamed himself for missing some of the physical signs of cardiogenic shock [shock from heart failure], and then he blamed the conditions under which he was expected to work: "You can't really do this job unless you get some rest. I stress rest because we're so tired we're not people, we're robots. You'd

be surprised how depressed cerebral function is when you're
really tired. And when you're here everyday thinking about
surgical problems, you don't notice other things. Look—I
know all the signs of heart failure. Christ, she was frothing at
the mouth. I'm sure she had pulmonary edema [filling of
lungs with fluid]. I know the signs, but they're not in the
front of my mind, you know, because I'm thinking about
pararectal abscesses [abscess adjacent to rectum], or wound
infections, and you don't always put together what is under
your nose. Today's thing, that's our fault. Last night she
should have had an emergency heart consultation, but it was
so late, we were so tired, we thought that it could wait until
morning" (Able Service).

Or subordinates claim that attendings' expectations are unrealistic and, if taken seriously, would require them to be in two
places at the same time:

Ernest and Josh were discussing the dressing-down Josh had
just received from Arthur and Grant. Josh repeated to
Ernest, who had missed rounds, a comment of Grant's that
attending rounds were for teaching but today so much
routine work had to be done, such as dressing changes, that
rounds had been a waste of everybody's time. Ernest told
Josh that this was probably the thing that pissed Arthur and
Grant off the most. Josh asked how the ward work could be
done if Arthur demanded that everybody be in the operating
room on surgery days. Josh mentioned that this morning they
had been down on the ward doing the scut only to get paged
so that they "could stand around and watch Arthur." Ernest
answered that as Josh knew it was Arthur's philosophy that
all housestaff be in the OR on surgery days, that even if
housestaff weren't actually doing the case they could learn
from watching Arthur. Ernest added that he thought
Arthur was right as far as that was concerned. Josh replied:
"Okay, then he shouldn't be pissed off if the work isn't
always done or if it was screwed up by some inexperienced
junior student." Ernest answered: "That's just the point.
Arthur assumed that since you weren't in the OR all day,
you were here doing the ward work. Look, you finished the

first case at 10:00 A.M. and you were in the second one
only from 11:30 to 1:00. So when the ward work wasn't
done, Arthur thought you were just goofing off" (Baker
Service).

Attendings accept no excuses when they decide that a subordinate shows them he has not been working hard enough to
meet minimal role requirements, to master the fundamentals
of patient care. Such subordinates are seen as simply not working hard enough, carefully enough, or seriously enough and
they are embarrassing the standards of patient care. Such
embarrassment is not gladly suffered by attendings; in fact, it
is not even tolerated. Yet it remains true that attendings spot
such lapses through a random check of behavior and then
generalize from it that an intern who does not even do this
must not be doing other things as well. This method of discovery keeps alive in subordinates the fear that a random and
unrepresentative event will cause them to be stigmatized. What
an attending sees and what he might see but does not notice is
the bedrock phenomena from which housestaff construct the
categories "good and bad luck." There are as a rule a number
of ways in which luck is not with the subordinate, and we have
outlined some of these above. There are also a number of ways
in which good fortune is with the subordinate, the ways in
work is organized to prevent an attending from noticing poor
performance. First, the subordinate rotates through a number
of services; this lessens the probability of substandard work
being spotted since each attending observes him for only a
short period (usually only eight weeks). Second, the corporate
nature of the service responsibility often means that those who
know what is going on may rescue those that do not. There is
the "filling in" that occurs during work rounds; and there is
the attending's practice of asking questions generally to the
group rather than directly to individuals.

   The first step of attending rounds, the first order of questions, establishes if subordinates are "on top of a situation,"
that is, if their organization of effort is meeting the basic

expectations of their superiors. The first level of questions discriminates subordinates into the worthy and the unworthy. Superordinates then move on to questions about the theoretical adequacy of the work done. This second level of questions rank-orders those who are considered worthy. At the second level of questioning, the attending shifts the focus from "what" to "why." He asks a subordinate to explain the reasons why he has done what he has done and what he hopes to effect by the course of his action. To an attending the subordinate's answer indicates his sophistication at medical reasoning. If the subordinate fails utterly, he may find himself back at the first-order questions. If the subordinate errs but indicates a grasp of the situation, the attending leads him through a reasoning exercise. Checks on reasoning may be made retrospectively or prospectively. Prospective checks are safest for attendings, patients, and housestaff. The reasoning exercises that attendings lead housestaff and students through is the way clinical expertise is passed on. This way of learning to make a diagnosis is one of the principal activities of clinical-medical education. For students and housestaff the process is the same: the examination of evidence and then a dialogue with the attending. In the episode below there are two such reasoning exercises: one of Arthur with Larry and one with Tom. Especially noteworthy is the quick and sarcastic way Larry is dismissed when he demonstrates that he does not know what is going on, as against the enthusiastic and almost collegial way Arthur expands Tom's suggestion:

We were in X ray. Arthur asked Tom, the senior student, "Do we have any interesting pictures for today?" "Just the consult from Gen Med." Arthur turned to a junior student: "Okay, Larry, what does this lesion suggest to you as your diagnosis?" "Ulcerative colitis?" Larry asked more than he answered. "Absolutely not. Try again." Larry suggests something weird. Arthur answers him: "I've only seen three cases of that in all my clinical experience! C'mon, think, will you! What did he get close to—a plane, and a propeller sliced off that portion of his colon? It's a tumor—I'm sure it's a cancer." Mark added: "On the diagnosis, you'd have to list it as

about eight and a half of the first ten possibilities." Arthur:
"Nine and a half. Okay, Tom, what should we do about it?
[A pause] Tom?" "I'm here. I was just thinking. I guess a left
colectomy or a total colectomy." Arthur: "This is a young
man. He's only thirty-eight. I think we should go for broke
and try to cure him. A total colectomy [total removal of colon
and rectum] and an ileostomy [an externalization of the lower
intestine]. We can cut it away and he can be cured and live
forty more years. Why be half-assed and risk recurrence?
This man's young. Is there any history of cancer in his
family?" Mark: "I don't believe so." "Then there is an eight
percent recurrence rate. That's pretty high, but it is much
higher with a history. This guy is only thirty-eight. It's really
unusual for cancer to appear in such a young guy—it's a real
tragedy. [To Grant] What a fascinating lesion! Let's put it
on the tumor clinic for Friday. It's tremendously unfortunate
for the patient, but it really is an interesting case. Poor
bastard" (Baker Service).

Moreover, this exchange also suggests an interesting ambivalence
of medical problems: namely, what is most exciting and interesting is often most tragic. By such interchanges clinical judgment is
formed. The subordinate suggests and the attending corrects. A
persistent and recurring problem then is the attending who corrects but neglects to give his reasons. Housestaff feel that this is
an abuse of rank.

There are several things to consider about controls at the
second level, or what I have called the "why?" level of questioning. First, mistakes at this level are assumed to be more correctable than mistakes at the first level. Second, the knowledge that
a subordinate's reasoning is flawed is apt to build slower than
first-level mistakes. Reasoning mistakes are seen as reflecting the
current state of a subordinate's art; it is harder for attendings to
see such mistakes as part of a pattern. Third, mistakes at the
second level do not engage as much of the subordinate's self in
the evaluation as mistakes at the first level. First-level mistakes
imply to attendings some sort of character defect. Second-level
mistakes imply only a lack of exposure to the proper material.

The Horror Story

As we have described them, the social controls established by
attending rounds are both flexible and harsh. They are harsh in
that the minimum standards set for acceptable work are quite
high and there are no acceptable excuses for not meeting these
standards. They are flexible in that once an individual has
demonstrated an ability and a willingness to meet these minimal,
albeit difficult, demands of the job, there are acceptable excuses
for error and mistakes. These mishaps become a routine part of
the environment and serve to reinforce a training definition of the
situation. We have described how the preeminence of clinical
expertise allows an attending to construct a binding interpretation of reality and how this power creates tensions among subordinates and between superordinates and subordinates. Now we
turn to one feature of social life among surgeons that tends to
dissipate everyday tensions to some degree—the horror story.

Horror stories, grotesque catalogs of all the things that can go
wrong in treating patients, abound in the hospital. From these
stories, we should not infer that hospitals deliver slipshod care;
rather, these stories should be seen as moral parables, an element
of the oral culture of medicine that remind all that healing is a
difficult business that must always be done with care. Evidence
that some horror stories may be apocryphal is the following: I
have heard different physicians-in-training in different types of
hospitals in different geographic regions repeat the same horror
stories. These stories have the quality of "just-so" tales: the
action is set in the past, exactly when no one can recall, and the
characters are persons whose names cannot be recalled. Horror
stories are told in two different ways. An attending may in the
course of events pass a story on to a subordinate. Attendings tell
three types of story. First is the cautionary parable:

> On attending rounds on Able Service, Peters asks: "What was
> this patient admitted with?" Carl answers: "Gastrointestinal
> bleeding in the emergency room." "And what did you do?"
> "Applied nasogastric suction and started an IV." Peters then

asks: "And where did these ministrations take place? In the
ER?" "On the floor." "Then you admitted the patient?"
Carl: "Why, yes, of course." Peters explains: "Well, that's
very important and shouldn't be taken for granted. Last
month, a friend of one of the staff went to the ER with
gastrointestinal bleeding and was sent home. He bled to
death. It's very important to remember to admit. What I'm
doing is keeping the lesson alive" (Able Service).

Of all horror stories, there are more variants of this than any
other I heard. In some versions, the "friend of the staff" is a
"visiting dignitary to the Pacific community." When housestaff
exchange the story among themselves, they invariably add that
the resident who treated the patient was dismissed the next
morning. The story drives home in a very concise way the need for
caution, care, and completeness. It allows an attending to communicate this by sharing a bit of hospital lore with his subordinate rather than by directly criticizing performance.

A second type of horror story that attendings exchange with
subordinates communicates the shared difficulties that they face
as surgeons:

Mark joined the Able Service late on rounds. As we left a
patient's room, White addressed him: "I hear you had some
problems up there [the operating room]." "Yeah. I couldn't
get the damn wound to stop oozing. I was getting pretty
aggravated. I thought that the anesthesiologists might have
given too much heparin [an anticoagulant]. But they had
written down one unit so I couldn't blame them." White
continued: "I figured something like that was happening
when you weren't down here. When I left you were ready to
sew her up. It is possible that the anesthesiologists gave too
much heparin. I once had a patient die that way. I once
ordered three units of heparin and the patient was mistakenly
given three ten-unit doses. So, instead of three thousand
units, he had thirty thousand units. We achieved some
hemostasis [stopping bleeding], but the patient died soon
after." Mark pointed out that "they don't keep those bottles
in the OR any more." "Yes, I know. I made a real big stink

downstairs and demanded that they all be removed" (Able
Service).

Such stories cataloging how the good work of surgeons at
Pacific is frustrated by others are quite common. Radiologists
and anesthesiologists are favorite targets, as are specialists in
internal medicine. The tales told about this latter group record as
a rule how their excessive caution and indecision prevent surgeons
from coming to the aid of patients until it is too late. Arthur is
able to recall numerous occasions when he was asked to consult
on patients in such advanced stages of disease that they were dead
within forty-eight hours. Another favorite source of such stories
are the surgeons at less prestigious hospitals who refer their
difficult problems to Pacific. The surgeons at Pacific even have
contemptuous terms for such physicians and their patients: the
physicians are LMDs (local medical doctors) and their patients
are "suburban specials." Mumford (1970) notes the same labeling phenomenon among the housestaff in the elite hospital she
studied. The surgeons at Pacific tell stories of how they have
received patients in the emergency room with no more information than "Pacific Hospital, Intensive Care" pinned to their
nightshirts. The dumps of others become horror stories:

> At one point on rounds, we stopped to discuss a patient
> referred from a hospital in a predominantly Jewish suburb.
> Arthur spoke: "That's one place that has killed more Jews
> than Eichmann. I can think of any number of atrocities
> committed there. Mr. Silver we salvaged through no fault of
> theirs. This one guy really pisses me off. He's been at at least
> two lectures where I've discussed the problem he sent us today
> and what does he do? An idiot stunt like taking out the
> appendix. That's like cutting down a tree to stop a forest
> fire. I can think of a few other patients he has killed. On one
> man, he removed most of the small bowel." "Jesus!" One
> student murmured. Arthur replied: "Yeah, that fellow met
> Jesus all right!" Rounds then continued (Baker Service).

Such stories circulate quite frequently. They are a way for surgeons to express open disapproval of behavior that they cannot

control. They are also, in an oblique way, defensive. The horror stories within the surgery department at Pacific occur for all to see; informing others of the disasters that happen elsewhere is a way for surgeons to claim: "What you see here may not be perfect, but it pales in comparison to what goes on elsewhere."

There is a third type of horror story that attendings tell their subordinates. This involves telling jokes on themselves. Between operations, in time-out periods, attendings recount the great adventures of their training. Such stories routinely recount their troubles with those surgeons who were their attendings. They indicate that attendings understand that mishaps are a normal part of training; that, indeed, such things have happened to them; and that they survived them. Moreover, the more off-color of these stories involve some conflict between duty and fun, usually symbolized by sex and alcohol. The values of a male culture are celebrated in locker-room language. Even in the tamest of such stories, the value of grace under pressure, profes- sional cool, is upheld:

> Toward the end of rounds, Arthur asked if anyone knew which island Hippocrates was from. When no one could answer, he turned to Grant and said: "Grant, it looks like you and I are the only two educated people on this service. Don't they teach you people any history of medicine?" Ernest answered that in his first year there were two noncredit lec- tures but he had been too busy to go. Grant stated that the history of medicine used to be studied if only to know the eponyms: "For instance, if you call something the 'Ernest syndrome,' the natural question is, 'Who is Ernest?'" Every- one laughed and Brian stepped forward: "We're laughing because we have discovered the 'Ernest syndrome.'" "Oh? What's that?" asked Arthur. "It's a patient with a left radical mastectomy who has a tattoo on the right contralateral thigh. It's named for Mrs. Fogg," answered Brian. Arthur laughed and added that during his training residents were given eponyms by attendings for stupid things that they had done: "For example, the Hammersmith phenomenon occurs when the resident cuts the attending's hand while removing the specimen. I remember when I got my eponym. I was doing my first total colectomy [total removal of colon and

rectum], with Dr. Cranz and he did it a little differently
than we do now. He clipped off the specimen with hemostats
[a small clamp]; he didn't tie it off the way we do now. Anyway, the specimen was out and I was bored sitting there
holding an idiot stick [a retractor] and the two other residents were removing hemostats from the specimen. They left
two on so I thought I'd be helpful and I reached up and
removed the hemostats just as the hemostat was perfectly
above the open wound and this liquid feces comes pouring
out. I thought to myself I'd better see when the first train
leaves for home. But Cranz didn't bat an eye. He just said,
'My, this is an unexpected development!' So he immediately
gets the sucker going to clean the wound. And he irrigated
the wound with a couple buckets of saline, and the operation
went on as if nothing had happened. The patient didn't bat
an eyelash recovering, and Dr. Cranz didn't say anything to
me until about a week after the patient left, when he said,
'You know, Arthur, that patient whom you performed the
intraperitoneal fecal lavage [an accidental washing of the
abdominal cavity with feces] on did very well.' So an intraperitoneal fecal lavage became known as the Arthur phenomenon" (Baker Service).

Needless to say, attendings do not tell such stories about themselves at the same time that they are dressing-down subordinates
for poor performance. Routinely, such stories are circulated after
an attending has "talked to" a subordinate and after the message has had some time to sink in. For the attending, telling a
horror story on himself is in a sense an attempt to reintegrate
both himself and his subordinates into a work group by matching
the humiliation he has forced on housestaff with some he willingly takes on himself. The second type of horror story on the
folly of others also has an integrative dimension since it includes
the auditor in the group of trusted people. As a general rule,
horror stories help transform outsiders into insiders by passing on
to them the secrets of the profession.

Horror stories are also told among subordinates themselves.
Here again the stories seem to fit one of three categories: (1)
directed against self, (2) directed against attendings, and (3)
directed against workers in the hospital. There are some routine

differences among the horror stories that attendings tell and the ones subordinates tell among themselves. First, the others that subordinates direct their stories against are usually lower-status workers in the hospital. Attendings never bother to tell stories about ancillary personnel. This reflects a difference between housestaff and attendings in whom they deal closely with: the point of the stories remains the same—those whom one relies on the most closely can destroy good work:

> On Able Service, a junior student told the following story that he had heard: A nurse's aide was assigned to watch a woman on a respirator. A patient at the other end of the hall had a cardiac arrest. The aide left the room to see what the commotion was about. The patient on the respirator turned her head and the tube kinked. By the time the nurse's aide returned, the cardiac monitor indicated a stopped heart. The patient was resuscitated but a vegetable. Three days later she died. The nurse's aide went undisciplined (Able Service).

> Today, Mr. Harmon claimed that he had been hurt by an X-ray technician in the ER and he asked for a shot of painkiller. As we left the room, Bill, the senior student, remarked that that technician had a reputation for being tough on patients. Bill said that when he was on a Gen Med rotation, a drunken man came in with a blow to the head. A subclavian line was inserted and X rays were ordered. At first, the technician refused to take the X rays. Then, when forced to, he treated the patient so roughly that he pulled out the subclavian and cracked the patient's ribs (Able Service).

A second difference between attending and housestaff horror stories concerns the way in which the stories are told. Subordinates circulate horror stories in a much more ritualized manner than do attendings. Two elements of story-telling practice are noteworthy. The stories themselves involve the sharing of various "firsts"—the first cutdown [entering a vein through an incision], the first proctoscopy [examination of rectum through a tube inserted into anus], the first intensive diagnostic study, and so on. These stories involve a catalog of all the things that can go wrong on the most routine procedure. In a sly way, these stories express an appreciation of and a sympathy for patients who provided early clinical experience:

> Stuart was telling us about his first intensive diagnostic study. He had noticed an abnormally low blood chemistry reading on a preadmission test. He showed the reading to the resident. For the next hour, he and the resident marched in and out of the patient's room asking about all sorts of strange diseases and symptoms. The patient became visibly nervous. Another blood test was given and the readings came back normal. Something had gone wrong in the computer (Able Service).

> We were talking outside the area where proctoscopies were done. Mark was telling us a story a friend had told him about his first proctoscopy. "He couldn't understand it. He couldn't get the proctoscope in at all. So he looks down and sees what he's done to this woman and without turning a hair he says, 'Well, that one is just perfect—great. Now hold on a few seconds longer while we get a look at the other opening down there'" (Able Service).

> Josh was retelling a story from his cardiac rotation: "It was the first time I was going to change a battery on a pacemaker. There was just me and this medical student in the OR and the patient had a cardiac arrest right after I put in the local anesthetic. I spent an hour and a half working on the guy while the anesthesiologist picked his nose. I was sure I was going to be out on my ass" (Baker Service).

Next, stories proceed in a one-up fashion and become increasingly more grotesque and macabre. Such story telling is an anteing-up of clinical credentials on the part of housestaff. Having a ready stock of stories serves notice that one has been around and knows what is going on.

The majority of stories that subordinates tell among themselves are directed against themselves. These stories serve a number of functions. First, like laughter, they relieve anxiety at the same time that they express it. This anxiety is usually over the fit between the person and the healer role. The highly ritualized form of the stories, especially the emphasis on inexperience, makes this anxiety all the more clear. Horror stories allow participants to communicate in a backhand way their awe at the tasks before them, their reverence for sound clinical judgment and experience, their apprehensions about the levels of their skills, and the secret knowledge that one learns from misadventure. Horror stories allow surgeons to comment on how ill the title "doctor" sometimes clothes the wearer. Second, horror stories allow guilt to be communicated and shared. These tales act to mitigate the strong norms of the role that prohibit physicians from expressing their feelings. Daniels (1961) presents a good discussion of how these norms are communicated in training. Third, horror stories are cautionary parables—they instruct the beginner that pride goeth before a fall.

Horror stories, then, are a recurring feature of behavior which helps mitigate the tensions of surgical training. By circulating secret knowledge such stories help recreate a sense of group after dressing-downs. As a rule, superordinates tell such stories for their heuristic value, but they also serve as a bit of comedy that relaxes tensions. Subordinates use these stories to establish their credentials as members of the group of surgeons. A repertoire of tales indicates a depth of experience. At the same time, horror stories allow access to affective dimensions of the self that normal fulfillment of the role denies. As such, they are a social control of the harsher aspects of ward rounds.

four

The Legitimation of Attending Authority

We have so far seen how failure is managed at the level of the work group. We have discussed the types of accounts that are given when deaths and complications occur, seen how these accounts are distributed throughout the division of labor, and shown how everyday routine surveillance acts as a means for superordinates to prevent and/or minimize failure and evaluate subordinate performance. Two features of this system of social control are noteworthy. First, knowledge of everyday performance is limited to members of the work group. Other colleagues do not observe each other's work and what information they do receive is systematically biased hearsay. That is to say, attendings, as well as housestaff, are most likely to grouse among themselves and spread information in those cases where they feel that the objective fact of a death or complication reflects unfairly on their performance.[1] The segregation of everyday controls and the great range of expressive behavior that attendings are allowed in applying them permits us to characterize such controls as private or backstage performances (Goffman 1961).[2] Second, the power of attendings in the system of everyday controls is truly remarkable. They alone decide if mistakes are forgivable or not, if subordinates are trustworthy or not. The binding understandings of failure forged at the everyday level are the attending's. His tolerance of technical and judgmental errors creates loyalty among subordinates and encourages greater efforts from them in the future to repay the obligation incurred by the attending's forgiveness. The swift and harsh dressing-downs that follow normative and quasi-normative errors define the boundaries within which forgiveness is permissible. Intolerance here creates rage and anger among subordinates and weakens ties to superordinates.

112

These two features of everyday controls—their privacy and the
extent of the attending's authority—arrest our attention, first for
their everyday operation and short-run consequences and second,
and even more important, because they seem to indicate that the
system of social control and socialization rests on an internal
contradiction. On the one hand, one overarching norm governs
the evaluation of performance, the rule of "no surprises"; full
and complete disclosures are demanded of subordinates. Yet, on
the other hand, superordinates are at an everyday level free of this
constraint. The privilege of their rank is that they need not
provide subordinates with any explanations for their actions. This
freedom from the constraint of full and complete disclosure is
what Weber defines as authority. Simply stated, this is the attending's power to give orders and expect that they will be carried
out. Earlier we have seen what beliefs attendings invoke to legitimate their treatment of subordinates, that is, to justify their use
of authority. What we have not yet explained is how attendings
maintain this considerable authority. This is not an unimportant
question, for authority does not just exist; its holders must take
great pains to maintain it against persons and events that challenge it.

In this chapter we shall explore the ways attendings dramatize
their claims to authority and hence maintain it. Such dramatizations are important for a number of reasons. To begin with,
they help explain the stability of attending authority. This stability should not be taken for granted, because when deaths and
complications occur the primary responsibility is the attending's.
Failure contradicts the attending's claim to powers beyond his
housestaff in a public and undeniable fashion. Furthermore,
these dramatizations explain what factors limit superordinate
authority and allow subordinates to accept it despite its occasional arbitrariness. Also, by displaying what norms attendings
must satisfy in order to maintain their legitimacy, they show how
attendings meet the requirements of full and open disclosure
that they demand of subordinates. Such dramatizations remind
everyone that attendings remain accountable for their actions and
go a long way toward resolving the contradiction between what

attendings require of their housestaff and what they require of themselves.

The attending's claims of authority rest first and foremost on external symbols independent of his day-to-day performance. These are his training, his experience, and his research contributions; however, such reputational assets would mean little if not reaffirmed by day-to-day performance. Therefore, attendings must both explain their failures—that is, they must neutralize or divest failures of their negative meanings—and they must also make their successes highly visible. The privilege of the attending's rank is not that he is free from accountability but rather that the forum in which his accounts for failure are demanded, given, and accepted is much more formalized, ritualized, and polite than the forum he provides his houseofficers and, further, he is provided a special forum to celebrate his successes. These two forums are the Mortality and the Morbidity Conference and Grand Rounds, respectively. Below we shall analyze both as occasions which attendings use to legitimate their claims to authority. In so doing, we shall see how paradoxically the harshness underlying the system of social control is at the same time mitigated and reinforced.

Varieties of Normal Action

In chapter 1 I stated that the presumption of success, which is the only warrant for subjecting a patient to the risk and trauma of an operation, makes surgeons more accountable than other physicians for failure. I claimed that the surgeon's craft and his beliefs about it make surgeons sensitive to what failure implies about their skill and judgment. In chapters 2 and 3 I examined how attendings held housestaff accountable for their actions. I am now in position to demonstrate how attendings transform the private troubles housestaff create for them into public issues in the Mortality and Morbidity Conference and Grand Rounds. Through these conferences attendings justify their claims to authority by public displays of virtuosity to the entire collegium of

subordinates and superordinates. The accounting of attending
surgeons is not a backstage activity but a very carefully staged
presentation of self. Subordinate accounting is always a test of
competence; superordinate accounting is always a display of
confidence.

As with all social accounts, those offered in the Mortality and
Morbidity Conference and Grand Rounds attempt to align discrepant outcomes and expectations. The possible relations among
any actions, expectations, and outcomes can be simply con-
ceptualized. To any action we attach either positive or negative
expectations; the action therefore either achieves or fails to
achieve its purposes. Merely for theoretic convenience are we
assuming that action in everyday life shares definitive endings with
dramatic action. Exactly when the curtain drops and the scene
ends is itself often an issue in everyday life. People express their
awareness of this by employing the following tactics to align
discrepant expectations and outcomes: they attempt to suspend
judgment and continue. They argue that the evidence is incomplete or that all the bugs in a plan are being worked out or, most
boldly, that success has already occurred but is not yet visible. A
good examination of this delaying tactic is found in Halberstam
(1972). Surgery, however, does not afford the same opportunities
as the Vietnam War for using this technique. The time horizon
for determining outcomes is restricted in surgery. This is one of
the features of the task-structure that makes surgeons so accountable. So, aware of the conceptual shortcomings involved, we can,
nevertheless, combine these two dimensions of action to form a
fourfold table that captures the possible relations among expectations and actions.

Action occurs in all cells, and groups evolve shared and patterned ways for treating such events. The more strained the fit of
expectations and outcomes, the more shared and patterned the
ways of treating them. The confusion and anxiety that occur when
things turn out other than the way we have planned need resolution. In such cases more elaborate structures evolve for explaining
the failure of our calculations than is the case when events

emerge as planned. In this table, cells 1 (expected success) and 4 (expected failure) represent no-confusion events. Expectations and outcomes are congruent. No elaborated ground rules are needed for actors to explain events. Relations are relaxed and there is great variation in interpersonal styles.

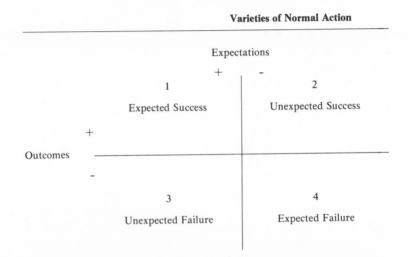

Varieties of Normal Action

Expectations

	+	−
1		**2**
Expected Success		Unexpected Success
3		**4**
Unexpected Failure		Expected Failure

Outcomes: +, −

Cells 2 and 3 are those in which more elaborate social accounting is necessary. These are confusing events. When an action turns out other than as planned it damns nothing so much as the power to diagnose a situation. Not surprisingly, the ability to diagnose a situation is something about which a physician cannot afford confusion. In the accounts offered to end this confusion, relations are formal and there is little variation in interpersonal styles. Cell 2 is unexpected success; accounting for it occurs in Grand Rounds. Cell 3 is unexpected failure; accounting for it occurs in the Mortality and Morbidity Conference, as well as at the everyday level that we described in chapters 2 and 3. As we shall see, the accounts offered in these two conferences differ substantially from those offered in the everyday face-to-face interaction among subordinate and superordinate.

No-Confusion Situations

Cell 1: Expected Success

In cell 1, where both expectations and outcomes are positive, we
have routine, unquestioned successful action. In surgery as in
everyday life, people do not ordinarily stop to question this action
or challenge those persons who achieve results.[3] Given the didactic component of clinical training, it is not entirely accurate to
state that attendings do not ask questions about routine and
ordinary successes. They do. However, they need not ask these
questions of their housestaff or of themselves. Routine success,
the happily removed appendix or the artfully repaired hernia,
threatens neither a houseofficer's nor an attending's credibility.
On the contrary, such success anchors their claims of expertise in
the empirical world and makes them substantial. However, such
success may create problems for the medical student. Since routine success does not compel the attending to exert time and energy
either keeping his subordinates in line or reexamining his own
decisions, he has more time for testing his student's knowledge.
Where the intern or resident is asked: "What went wrong?"
"How did this happen?", the student is asked: "Why did this
work?" "Why did we choose this course of action rather than
some other?" Routinely such questioning is not very intense. The
student serves as a convenient foil for the attending. Since this
rotation is the student's first exposure to surgery, attendings do
not always expect correct answers to such questions. Attendings
use such questioning to expose and to impress on students their
ignorance, to demonstrate the intellectual rigor needed for the
surgical management of disease, and to illustrate some general
principles of surgery.[4] Thus, even though routine and expected
success may make an occasional student uncomfortable, it does
not create confusion about what is going on. Colleagues do not take
excessive notice when one simply meets the expectations of
others. Only the most professionally infantile, the students, are
invited to speculate about why success occurred. There is a parallel
here to parents who ask children how simple objects work in order

to demonstrate some simple causal relationships. Those initiated into a social world no longer wonder how such things work. They take them for granted. Action that falls in cell 1 ratifies the tacit assumptions on which surgery rests. It is not a topic for social accounting; rather, it is the background from which accountable events emerge.

Cell 4: Expected Failure

Cell 4, in which expectations and outcomes are negative, contains cases for which no elaborate social accounting is necessary. Patients who are hopelessly ill with terminal diseases fall into this category. What happens to these patients, although tragic, could not have been otherwise. According to Fox (1974), attitudes toward the discussion of the practical, existential, and ethical issues surrounding the care of the dying patient have changed considerably in medical schools over the last twenty years. What was formerly dismissed as merely philosophical is now openly discussed. In surgery, as in other areas of medicine, there is a concern for the humane treatment of dying patients. This enlarged discussion indicates a greater sensitivity on the part of medical educators to the fact that expected failure can be a trial on the personal and individual level at the same time that it is a normal event in a professional life. With the increased healing power of modern medicine there has arisen the need to make more explicit the individual strategies for handling the question, How do I recognize when a situation is hopeless and then what do I do? Confusion exists in this situation, to be sure, but this confusion is of a different order than that of cells 2 and 3, where expectations and outcomes are discrepant. The confusion that surrounds the hopeless cases of cell 4 is existential and individual. In cells 2 and 3, confusion is social and scientific. The difference is this: in cell 4, the physician must account for why an individual patient developed an untreatable cancer that both he and the patient would have preferred not to occur. In cell 2, he must account for how he salvaged an incurable. In cell 3 he must account for how he lost a curable. There is here a question of

responsibility. Cells 2 and 3 clearly raise questions of professional
responsibility. Cell 4 is at the boundary between individual and
human responsibility and professional responsibility. To help
their subordinates deal with the problems raised by the hopeless
cases of cell 4, attendings pass on to housestaff and students their
beliefs about when and how a patient should be allowed to die:

> We reached Mr. Starvos's room on rounds. We paused a long
> time before his door. Nothing was said. Everyone looked at
> the ceiling or down at the floor. Eye contact among people
> was not established. Finally Arthur said: "Goddammit." It
> was the group's signal to enter the room. Mr. Starvos com-
> plained of pain. He was alert and lucid. We left quickly.
> Arthur spoke: "He's too damned alert—that's all there is to
> it. Look, I'm not one to give up on patients but we have to
> realize that there comes a time when we can do nothing more
> for a patient and we should no longer support life but the let
> the patient die comfortably with as much dignity as pos-
> sible. In all honesty I think we have to admit we've reached
> that point with Mr. Starvos. He's too alert for that much
> pain. He shouldn't be that awake. Let's begin to give him
> Librium and morphine. Yeah—Librium and MS [mor-
> phine]—that should make him more comfortable. Mark, first
> talk to his wife. Make sure that his will is in order, all his
> bank accounts are square, and the property straight away.
> Then begin the Librium and MS. He's too alert. He needs
> sedation. Also, are they Catholic or Greek Orthodox? His
> wife was asking about a priest—I think it's time to tell her to
> bring him in. We can't do any more for him." The group
> saw one more patient on rounds and then Arthur mentioned
> Starvos again: "Look, there comes a time when you have to
> acknowledge your limits and make the patient as comfortable
> as possible. I think we can discontinue monitoring his vital
> signs at night. There's no reason to wake him up in the
> middle of the night to take his temperature, pulse, blood
> pressure, and all that other bullshit. Let's close the door,
> leave him with his family, and let him die with some dignity,
> as a man instead of a patient with a glass tube up his ass.
> We've done what we can. Let him die, poor man" (Baker
> Service).

On rounds, Arthur was discussing proper care of the dying
patient. "You can't offer these patients shit but you have to
go in there and perform a laying-on of hands, so to speak.
You can't abandon them." The service had just visited a consult on the medical service and Arthur had decided that the
patient's cancer was too advanced to warrant an operation.
He continued: "That patient is terminal. Let's send her home
with morphine and Librium and let her be with her family.
If it was your mother, would you want her in the hospital?
Remember that Chinaman they wanted us to operate on last
week? He died forty-eight hours later. Christ, you could look
at him and see that he was half dead—the medicine people
said, 'No, it's because he's Chinese and they all look like
that.' They'd be hanging IV's into their patients all the way
to the morgue if we'd let them" (Baker Service).

There are, of course, grave differences of opinion on when it is
the "proper time" to allow a patient to die with dignity. Surgeons
are not known for throwing in the towel quickly. Nurses and
physicians in other specialities are often critical of what they
consider needless surgery, claiming that it extends suffering
rather than life. Moreover, as a rule, subordinates are quicker
than superordinates to decide that a patient is beyond help, a fact
which is possibly more a comment on their control of treatment
and their investment in its correctness than in their personal
philosophies. But this is all quite beside the point: when it is
expected, death threatens neither the professional self of the
subordinate nor of his superior. One of the hard lessons that one
must learn in surgery, as in all branches of medicine, is that there
are times when nothing more remains to be done. Again, colleagues do not need to account when the unsalvageable are not
salvaged. Action that falls into cell 4, like that which falls into cell
1, ratifies the tacit assumptions that make action in a scene
possible, although these assumptions are of a different order.
Action in cell 1 underscores how much suffering surgery is able to
alleviate. Action in cell 4 points to the limits of surgery. It
indicates how much is beyond the surgeon's skill and knowledge.
Routine success and routine failure both have an air of inevit-

ability which renders accounting unnecessary and which makes the extraordinary success or failure all the more conspicuous.

Confusing Situations

In terms of the sheer volume of cases, most action falls in cells 1 and 4. Cases in cells 2 and 3, unexpected success or failure, is much more rare. Because of their scarcity, these are professional events of some importance and at Pacific—as at most teaching hospitals—special ceremonies for the entire congregation of surgeons have evolved for witnessing them, resolving the confusion they create, and incorporating them into the group's history and the individual's biography. The fact that the marking of unexpected success or failure is a group ceremony of special importance is indexed by two facts. First, the two conferences in which they are discussed—Grand Rounds and the Mortality and Morbidity Conference—are the only occasions when all ranks and subgroupings of the Department of Surgery gather. And, second, they are the only occasions when work groups will put off tasks at hand—save operating, drop whatever they are doing, and attend a conference. As others have noted (Miller 1970), the houseofficer is faced with the dilemma of having to attend numerous confernces and provide patient care. The demands of both on his time cannot be satisfied and the individual adopts a short-run perspective which allows him to get by: he provides patient care and skips conferences. I also found this pattern—except for Grand Rounds and the Mortality and Morbidity Conference where the individual's normal accommodation is reversed. In surgery, all conferences wait until work is done, save these two. This is true for all ranks of the hierarchy. Attendings, as well as their underlings, feel compelled to attend and be on time. This punctual assembly of those accustomed to letting others cool their heels is quite remarkable. Schwartz (1974) has discussed waiting as an index of power of persons. Here punctuality testifies to the power of events.

What interests us about these meetings is the role attendings play in them. Attendings use these meetings to demonstrate their clinical wisdom which, as we noted, underlies their authority. The arbitrary elements of quick decisions justified only by rank and contradicted at times by scientific evidence are mitigated. By reserving for himself the right to resolve confusion, the attending legitimates his authority in these forums. The fact that unexpected success allows this is hardly surprising. However, that they are able to transform the negative experience of an unexpected failure into a positive one that serves as evidence of their wisdom is surprising and in need of some explanation. For the moment, suffice it to say that this satisfies the demands of the "heroic" element of the surgical role. The hero takes credit for his success but he is also able to accept the responsibility for his failures, to admit them openly, and to seek to remedy them. Through his trials, the hero learns the value of humility. As we have seen at the subordinate level, those who cannot behave with proper humility are seen as normatively wanting. This is also true at the attending level. In the following discussion of Grand Rounds and the Mortality and Morbidity Conference, we shall see how attending performance legitimates the application of everyday controls and how attendings use both meetings to demonstrate that they are worthy of the mantle of leadership since they accept its burdens along with its rights and privileges.

Cell 2: Unexpected Success—Grand Rounds

Grand Rounds celebrate the extraordinary successes of surgeons in cases where expectations are negative and outcomes are positive. In cell 2 of our chart we have ground-breaking success, such stuff as medical journal articles are made of. As we stated earlier, surgeons do not ordinarily operate with negative expectations. However, there are certain circumstances in which the presumption of success is suspended. Most commonly, two conditions make waiving the presumption of success warrantable. First, it is acceptable to waive the presumption of success when surgery is the only alternative left for a patient and it offers some hope, however slim, of salvaging the patient. Such situations inform the notion of the surgeon as hero.[5] Less glorious are cases where the patient's condition intersects with the surgeon's research interests. At such times the surgeon rules out alternatives quicker than usual and operates. Colleagues appreciate the courage, judgment, and skill necessary to succeed in these situations. Grand Rounds allow them to express this appreciation. Grand Rounds also allow each attending the chance to demonstrate that good reasons exist for the tyranny of his clinical judgment.

At a group level, Grand Rounds allow the entire collegium to review the most recent successes of their colleagues and beyond that the generalizable principles that are emerging for the surgical management of disease. As a weekly ritual, Grand Rounds reconfirm for everyone that Pacific deserves its national reputation for excellence. At an individual level, Grand Rounds provide attendings an arena to display their virtuosity. When questioned about why they chose careers in academic medicine, attendings invariably mention the importance of peer recognition:

> When I started medical school, I had the desire to be a
> surgeon. Surgeons were the most impressive guys, they got a
> lot of attention, they always seemed to be doing things. And
> I had a desire for all this; but the decision comes later when
> you graduate from medical school and you have all the train-
> ing before you. The training comes in two phases. In
> England, they are kept quite distinct, but here they are often
> intermingled. In the first phase, you must simply learn
> surgery: you have to learn techniques, pick up the basics. In
> the second phase, you have to learn judgment; you have to
> learn when to operate, when not to, and what operations to
> perform. And then when you finish, you have to decide if
> you're happy with this status or not. Now the "true" doctors
> who serve a community and are content to perform the
> common operations for the common conditions stop here.
> But there are those of us dissatisfied with this status who go
> into academic medicine. We want to do things that others
> can't. We want all the difficult cases referred to us. We want
> to train others to be good surgeons. We want to be recog-
> nized by our colleagues as an expert on some problem
> (Attending).

> Well, there are two aspects to that. One is, it's a real ego trip.
> You're surrounded by a small nucleus of people; and you're
> always patting each other on the back, telling each other how

great you are. Sometimes it's nothing more than a group of men playing children's games ... the support of the peer group makes up for the financial sacrifices. So it's really a supportive atmosphere. It's gratifying to be at the top of the profession and have people tell you how good you are all the time. Second, although there are a lot of advantages to being in private practice—you can make more money, you can come home earlier, you have more free time—it can be very boring. You don't get the most interesting cases and you're surrounded by a lot of crap. Doctors who let patients die because they think that cancer is always incurable. You can really go out of your mind watching people practice bad medicine because they don't know any better. But here you can practice medicine in the highest quality circumstances. It's an ego trip. You pay heavily for it in terms of salary, administrative nonsense, long hours, family life, and personal life and leisure. A lot of it is really childish stuff but a lot of it feels really good. It's an ego trip to handle the toughest cases, to challenge yourself, and be among the best (Attending).

Grand Rounds provide an itinerary for the attending's ego trip; this conference assures that the peer recognition that attendings desire is provided in a fairly regular fashion. This recognition of skill comes in a much more direct and personal way than research publications provide. Of course, there are many other ways that colleagues pay homage to each other's skill. Informal consultation is one. More dramatic is when an attending acts as his colleague's first assistant. Here, he willingly subordinates himself to his equal, merely for the opportunity to watch the other work. Given the crowded nature of the attending's workday, such tributes are rare. When they occur, they highlight an aesthetic appreciation of flawless technique. Regularly scheduled, Grand Rounds are a device to distribute the amount of formal colleague support, approval, and recognition equitably. The rotation of the one to three cases presented weekly at Grand Rounds among services helps guarantee that the distribution of peer support is at least formally equal, despite whatever inequities evolve in the methods that colleagues informally grant approval.[6] Grand Rounds then serve to legitimate attending authority by demonstrating the high regard that attendings have for one another. For attendings, this regard is one of the primary rewards of the work environment.

More important, Grand Rounds allow attendings to model for their subordinates the proper way to accept their place in the medical elite. At the same time, this modeling is done in such a fashion to dramatize for subordinates the distance they must travel during training before they can claim to be equals. The standards of decorum that govern case presentation, the complete presentation of the clinical history, the review of the relevant literature, the elegant technique amply illustrated by slides of the operation, and their own restricted roles in the proceedings—all impress on subordinates the seriousness of the tasks before them, the accomplishments of their superordinates, and their own insignificance in bringing about these miraculous results. Grand Rounds model the virtuous performance of virtuous performance. The recurrent, almost invariant, mode of case presentation makes this modeling specific. First, subordinates present the clinical history of the patient. A good performance by a subordinate is one that as clearly and concisely as possible recounts an involved, complex clinical history. The subordinate gives a simple report, something which is not always a simple task. The subordinate is then for all practical purposes finished. He sits down and the superordinate takes over. First, the superordinate clarifies any ambiguity that arose during the subordinate's account. He then interprets the case history just presented. This interpretation routinely comprises a review of the clinical literature, a review which indicates that the attending's method for handling the case can improve the current mortality and morbidity rates. He adumbrates general principles which indicate that his results are replicable for all who would correctly apply his techniques.

But for one digression from professional and technical demeanor such an order of events would be entirely unremarkable. During the change of actors from subordinate to superordinate and the change of action from narration to interpretation the patient is often brought in and displayed for the group. Now, in some cases such as orthopedic ones, where the lame are literally made to walk, such presentations make sense; in most instances, however, the purpose is less clear as the group witnesses nothing more than a closed scar. The patient is asked a few questions about how he used to feel and how he feels now. Then he is led out. Once the patient is removed to the wings, the attending begins his exposition of the case. He renders a technical and learned account of the success. Case presentation lasts from thirty to forty-five minutes. The patient is present for generally less than three minutes.

These interruptions in what is for the most part very highly technical talk are striking for their brevity and their superficiality. Housestaff and attendings make jokes about the practice and complain that it serves no discernible purpose and that they learn nothing from it. Yet, if this is the case, why is this practice so regularly adhered to and why in those cases in which it is forgone is the attending presenting the case likely to include in his slide presentation a smiling snapshot or two of his cured patient?[7] First and most concretely, the patient is a living testimonial to the validity of the claims being made. Second, the interview with the patient shows the attending surgeon at his humanistic best. It allows him to demonstrate that alongside the technical expert about to teach a lesson, there is a humane healer who deals with the patient as a person. Third, the presence of the patient is gratifying for the attending. He is displaying one of the achievements he is most proud of, and he is in turn praised by his colleagues for this. Fourth, the introduction of the patient in the middle of the discussion reinforces group commitments by showing a case when the limits of the possible were extended. The whole group can share the sense of worthiness such patients inspire. The proud display of patients is a striking feature of Grand Rounds; however, display is limited to this conference. When patients who fall into cell 2 return to the clinic for follow-up visits, attendings round up as many subordinates and colleagues as possible for "ad hoc" displays:

I was in the clinic with Josh and Brian. They were writing charts in the work area when Arthur came in and told us all to go to examining room "D." There, Josh, Brian, and I were introduced to a patient. Arthur recited a brief history and invited an examination of his patient. Josh and Brian quickly examined the patient, nodded appreciatively, and then went about their tasks. Arthur thanked the patient and we left the room together. In the work area he turned to me and said: "That's why we're so demanding around here. By all rights that man should be dead. But there he is. That's the edge you get when you really bust your hump." He whistled to himself as he wrote a progress note in the patient's chart (Baker Service).

Finally, the last remark of Arthur's alerts us to what may be the most important feature of patient presentation. The display of past successes is an irrefutable argument to subordinates for the attending's hegemony. It is as if by this practice the attending tells his subordinate: "We can talk as equals when you have results like this to show off. Until then, respect the experience that achieves such results." Such displays of patients dramatize the distance between attendings and housestaff who do not have a ready stock of miraculous cures to parade.

Grand Rounds legitimate an attending's authority by dramatizing his most spectacular successes. Skill at presenting such cases is known as "roundsmanship"; it is a much appreciated skill. Those who have it are able to make the most of their extraordinary successes; and it is such ability that builds surgical reputations. Surgeons demonstrate this ability by elegantly explaining the extraordinary. Such performances dramatize the distance between them and their subordinates who, for whatever private praise they are given, are only allowed a very minor role in the proceedings.

Cell 3: Unexpected Failure—The Mortality and Morbidity Conference

It is not surprising that attendings use their extraordinary successes to legitimate the rigid hierarchical authority system of a surgical service. It is, however, noteworthy that they are able to use unexpected failure to serve the same end. In this section we explore the transformation of negative evidence into a positive display of an attending's skill. This transformation occurs in the Mortality and Morbidity Conference, in which cases that fall into cell 3—where expectations are positive and outcomes are negative—are discussed. The Mortality and Morbidity Conference is a form of retrospective peer review. The fact that attendings are able to use this forum to further consolidate their claims to authority is all the more remarkable when we consider that in this forum the attending's failures are presented for all to see and that this is the only occasion in surgical training that exists for public and open criticism of attending surgeons.

In the Mortality and Morbidity Conference the private understandings of failure achieved at the everyday level (chapters 2 and 3) are transformed into public knowledge. This transformation consists by and large of purging from the accounts the categories of normative and quasi-normative error and with them the implications of careless, lazy, negligent, or insubordinate performance they carry. At the Mortality and Morbidity Conference failure is accounted for professionally, that is, the reasons presented for it—with one notable exception—are formal and technical. In a sense this fact alone increases the power of the attending and further obligates his housestaff since the attending allows the knowledge of such substandard performance to remain a form of private, albeit guilty, knowledge.[8] Four factors account for the omission of normative and quasi-normative errors from discussion. First, such errors are an implicit indictment of an attending's control of his staff so it would ill serve him to publicize them. Second, attendings believe that if a subordinate makes a normative or quasi-normative breach on one service, he is likely to make them on others. There is no need to publicly humiliate subordinates; events will do so soon enough. Third, these errors are seen as indicative that unfit subordinates have character or personality disorders. There is little profit from exposing them since there is little hope of correcting them. Fourth, one purpose of the Mortality and Morbidity Conference is to illustrate that failure and error are an inevitable part of surgery and the best that one can hope for is to learn from these unfortunate hap-

penings so as not to be condemned to endlessly repeating them.
To introduce the scolding that accompanies normative and quasi-
normative errors into the Mortality and Morbidity Conference
would only encourage attempts to conceal complications. The
metapurpose of the conference would be destroyed if failure were
not treated as matter of factly as possible.

Like Grand Rounds, the Mortality and Morbidity Conference
has a remarkably consistent structure. However, the proceedings
have one more degree of freedom than do Ground Rounds, and it
is a very significant one. At the beginning of the meeting an
agenda is circulated. [9] The agenda lists the order of case presentation. The agenda provides the following information for each
case: the patient's age and sex, the service responsible for him,
the preoperative diagnosis, the procedures performed, and the
reason for presentation at the conference (either death or a specific complication). Also on the agenda is a record of the number
of major and minor operations performed by each service in the
preceding week. The agenda is a box score, and case presentation
is the play-by-play commentary. Case presentation is similar to the
format of Grand Rounds. The subordinate begins and gives a
case history. However, his job does not end here. He is on stage to
answer questions about the propriety of his behavior until either
his superordinate steps forward to give an interpretation of the
clinical history and an explanation of nodal choices, or until
another superordinate directs a question to his colleague. This
option of the attending to step forward or not is the degree of
freedom that the Mortality and Morbidity Conference possesses
that Grand Rounds do not. It is the exercise and use of this option
that allows attendings to transform a conference ostensibly about
their failure into a forum to celebrate their authority. We shall
now see how this is so.

The cases that are presented at the Mortality and Morbidity
Conference can be described in four basic ways. These are the
"normal troubles" of surgery. Each of these has its own accounting strategy. Two are relatively straightforward and do not
involve the attending playing a role in the proceedings unless
forced to. Two are relatively more complex and involve the at-

tending taking an active role in the accounting. In the first two cases it would be beneath the attending's dignity to explain failure where the causes are painfully obvious. In the latter two cases it would be beyond the houseofficer's skill to explain the failure, interpret the attending's strategy, and determine why events took the untoward turn they did.

The first and most simple case is when there is a routine complication easily managed after surgery. The complication is resolved without incident and, aside from the complication, the patient's recovery is uneventful. An example of such a case is a wound infection. For such cases accounting is as a rule solely the subordinate's responsibility.[10] Subordinates in this case align expectation and outcome by the claim that when all factors are taken into account—factors that were by their very nature unknowable before surgery—the outcome is really a success. The case belongs in cell 1 of our fourfold table. The argument that the complication notwithstanding the surgery was in fact a success hinges on the following claims: that although the rate of complication is known for a population at large, any individual occurrence cannot be predicted; that in this case sound prophylactic techniques have been applied but to no avail; and that once the complication presented itself, it was routinely and successfully treated. Such cases do not greatly arrest the attention of the conference's participants. So long as the subordinate clearly presents the case and competently answers a few questions, the case is quickly dispatched. Competently answering questions here means demonstrating that one knows what went wrong and why and that one has learned a lesson from this experience. The superordinate need not step forward since the patient's recovery as well as the thoughtful performance of his subordinate indicates that he is well aware of the situation and has it under control. The complications that are easily and quickly resolved are the ones that concern surgeons least, both in formal peer review and in everyday social control. In either circumstance, they are not seen as threats to competence but rather as routine and calculable parts of the environment.

The second straightforward case is the terminally ill patient and the questions his treatment provokes. When such patients are operated on, it is usually to palliate the more gruesome aspects of disease or to make a heroic attempt to rescue a trauma victim. The tactic of interpretation here is to have the expectation of success waived. The subordinate claims that the only reason that the service operated was because the situation provided no alternative, save the speedy signing of a death certificate. He claims that had the surgery been successful a miracle of modern medicine would have occurred. The case would have fallen into cell 2 of our table and have been appropriate for discussion at Grand Rounds. But since nothing of the sort happened, the patient was really without hope, and the case belongs to cell 4.

Straightforward as this accounting strategy is, it is not as readily acceptable to superordinates as the first tactic of interpretation outlined above. This is understandable if for no other reason than that death rather than recovery is the outcome in need of explanation. There are certain situations in which this accounting strategy is easily accepted by the audience. For example, there is the case of the trauma victim who receives multiple injuries and whose life is mechanically supported until the family decides if they will allow the cadaver to donate organs.[11] Another example is a patient operated on previously for the palliation of cancer's more gruesome sequelae who is successfully discharged and returns to the hospital some months later for terminal care because the family can no longer provide supportive care at home. Now, for such patients, ethical and philosophical questions may be raised: Did intervention add to or subtract from the patient's suffering? What is the relationship between the technical expertise we may demonstrate as surgeons and our humane responsibilities as healers? Though such questions are raised, they routinely serve to end discussion rather than begin it. In fact, those who raise questions about whether an operation was necessary or not often note that these questions are philosophical and inappropriate since the action has already occurred. Surgeons have a studied dislike for discourse on philosophical questions. They define such questions as endlessly debatable and, with their action ethic, surgeons have an almost trained incapacity to debate questions without answers. This is all the more so in cases where the patient's death is a certainty. Surgeons view debate here as unprofitable because "we know that exit is assured and all we would really be talking about is the mode" (Mortality and Morbidity Conference). Philosophic and ethical questions in this context signal members of the conference that, from the viewpoint of surgery as a scientific and value-free activity, they have nothing more to discuss. Moreover, attendings resist public discussions about the necessity of surgery and for good reasons. They fear publicly accepting any general principles for the limitation of effort. The internalization of such principles by the lazy, the unprincipled, or the inexperienced would, they feel, dilute the quality of care and provide an overly broad rationale for less than committed care. Noteworthy here is the contrast between the public silence of attendings at the conference and their private speech backstage on rounds about the limits of care and the treatment of the dying.

There are two situations in which the questions usually raised to end discussion begin it. The first of these is very rare. Attendings explain those cases which by all rights should have been the miraculous cures of cell 2, but which they chose instead to treat as the hopeless cases of cell 4. So extraordinary is such an event that it is set off from normal proceedings by the fact that the superordinate handles the presentation himself. He gives both the narration and exposition. He takes total responsibility. The subordinate plays no role in the proceedings at all.

Dr. Porter, a pediatric surgeon, stepped forward to present the third case himself, mumbling as he walked to the front of the room, "I think I'd better take care of this myself." He began: "This third case is very different from the first two presented. Where the first two cases involve questions of patient selection and the taking of risk to prolong life, cases where everything must go right if the surgical intervention is to succeed, this third case involves the taking of risk not to prolong life. This is a decision that only an attending physician

can make and for which he alone is responsible. This infant
was born with 'prune belly' [wrinkling of skin on the belly
from absence of abdominal muscles], complete atresia of
the urethra [closing of outflow from urinary bladder], various
deformities of the legs and feet which may have been the
result of the fetus's position and may have been corrected
with time, an omphalocele [a large hernia at the umbilicus],
and a heart murmur. The obstetrician and the pediatrician
at the hospital where the infant was born put the baby aside
to die; but, as luck would have it, it did not. They then called
me up to arrange a transfer. They both expressed the hope
that the baby would die, but in my hands. Here is where the
situation gets complicated. The mother is a thirty-year-old
woman. She married at twenty-six and put off conception a
number of years while she was under psychiatric care. Then
she had some trouble conceiving and finally she had this
baby. She had never seen the child. The father, acting with
the obstetrician and the pediatrician, had arranged the
transfer and supported the decision not to make heroic efforts
to save the child's life. I thought we had to be straightforward
enough in this case to inform the mother of the baby's
problems and its chances because of the psychological
aspects of the mother-child, mother-father, doctor-patient
relationship, as well as our various legal responsibilities. So
I did the minimum necessary to give the baby a chance until
the mother could see it. I repaired the omphalocele. The
mother did come up and see the baby. She was obviously
under heavy sedation and quite difficult to deal with. She
waxed and waned in her support of the child. She couldn't
decide if the baby should survive. It was then that I decided
that the baby should not be considered for cardiac arrest
treatment, and that no urgent or emergency measures should
be taken to save the baby's life. These children need total
support if they are to have any chance at all. This baby would
never be normal and without the total support of both
parents there was no hope for a satisfactory adjustment. I
have seen many marriages totally disrupted by the extensive
hospitalization that such cases require after a number of
years. This is why I decided to let the infant die. This is, as
I said before, a decision that only an attending can make. It

is needless to say a very difficult decision. Yet in this case it is one that I'm totally comfortable with" (Mortality and Morbidity Conference).

After this presentation, no questions were asked. The attending's right to make this decision and his grounds for doing so remained unexplored. Rare as these cases are, they do establish what considerations are used to establish the boundaries of effort. Interesting here is the surgeon's definition of his client as the entire family network; his interpretation of the Hippocratic injunction, "First, do no harm"; and his weighing the quality of life against the mere fact of life itself. The very extraordinariness of this set of circumstances and the attending's public account of his decision making show how firmly embedded the principle is that the surgeon must do everything possible to prolong life.

This brings us to the second set of circumstances in which the attempt to assign patients to cell 4 as a hopeless case raises rather than ends questions for the audience. Here, the audience questions the subordinate's interpretation that the patient was in fact a hopeless case. They challenge the subordinate's interpretation of the case as inevitable death. Such challenges are likely to bring attendings in conflict with one another since it was the attending in charge who more likely than not made most of the management decisions with regard to the case and who has discussed the cause of death and the case's presentation with the subordinate onstage and on-the-spot at the moment:

Andrew, a resident, had just explained that the death of an elderly lady following a gallbladder removal was caused by her old age and general physical weakness. He was immediately challenged by an attending. "That's not what I would call thinking real hard. I mean, you didn't exactly scratch your head until it bled on this one, did you, Andrew? You can't stand there and tell us this lady died from old age. If she was going to die from old age, why operate on her to begin with?" Dr. White, the attending on the case, rose to his resident's defense: "You're not exactly being fair. You know well enough that things like this can happen any time. It was just one of those unpredictable catastrophes." The other

attending answered: "That's bullshit. It doesn't sound like the
treatment of this lady was very well thought out." White
replied, "C'mon now, you have your share of cases like this.
She was a very strange old woman" (Mortality and Morbidity
Conference).

The attending's defense of his subordinate is a defense of
himself and his control over events. Beyond that, the attending
rescues the houseofficer from an uncomfortable situation. In so
doing he repays the subordinate for the indignities he subjects
him to in everyday situations. Such defenses are evidence of the
attending's authority and how it is used to shield as well as attack
subordinate performance.

You have to remember when something bad happens it's
usually at my instigation. Now, my orders may not have been
properly carried out. I may have ripped into the resident
before M&M. But I'm the responsible agent and I have to
back up my own people. You can't allow yourself to fall into
the syndrome of everything-that-goes wrong-is-the-resident's-
fault (Attending).

While disagreements may become as heated as the one above,
this rarely happens. The attending's support of his subordinate
and his assurance that everything possible was done is usually sufficient to quiet debate. So, despite the perturbations described
above, the strategy of having some failures redefined as cases that
fall into cell 4 is accomplished easily enough. This may be a
self-protective mechanism operating among attendings, an operative norm of reciprocity: if nobody pushes too hard, nobody will
be pushed too hard. Further, pushing too hard challenges the
deeply ingrained norm of individual responsibility for the patient
and is an affront to the decorousness of relationships among
colleagues.

The majority of the cases discussed at the Mortality and
Morbidity Conference are dispatched by the two tactics of interpretation discussed above. However, accounting for some failure
is relatively more complex. In these cases, the attending plays a
very important role in the proceedings and this role is an addi-

tional method for legitimating his authority. There are two types of problems that require this more complex method of social accounting.

In the first of these, surgeons must choose from among a number of procedures, none of which particularly recommend themselves. The probability of success for procedure A is the same as for procedure B or C and is in any case uniformly low. The surgeon must account for the procedure chosen when there are no clinically established protocols for it or any other procedure. These are the procedures that attendings at Pacific perform in order to maintain their standings as members of the national elite. Such cases are very important to attendings, they are evidence of their special place in medicine. Failure here disturbs the assumption that the attending's pride of place is deserved. This pride of place is, by the way, not a tacit background assumption but is right at the foreground of social consciousness, a constantly reiterated and well-articulated part of the work environment:

> The nurses on Baker Service were having problems with a patient. He was, in their opinion, irascible and they said they were tired of his addressing them in abusive tones. They complained to Dr. Grant, claiming it was not so much the patient's requests as the way he made them that bothered them. Dr. Grant answered: "Look—we will not put with this. We have all been under a lot of strain lately. You girls have been working particularly hard and we do not have to put up with an abusive patient. The way I look at it, we are doing Mr. Jameson a favor by operating on him—no other hospital around here would. He is an extremely poor operative risk. We do not promise our patients first-class hotel accommodations when they come here, nor do we promise them excellent cuisine. We only promise to get them better when no one else will treat them. It is we who are doing them a favor and not they us. This is really the same thing we went through with Michael Chometz. I'll talk with Mr. Jameson. And if he doesn't like what I say, then—fine! That is one less headache for us all" (Baker Service).

Arthur had just operated on the wife of a close friend—her prognosis was poor, and he was complaining to me (he had

steered me to a corner where we were alone). "In academic
medicine you're motivated by the desire to be the best. That
means that you do a lot of cases that no one else would touch,
and that a lot of friends send their families to you. And while
I really hate the work, I'd hate it more if they thought someone else was better and they went to him. It's tough treating
these problems. Son of a bitch, it's the toughest part of
practice" (Baker Service).

Earlier, we noted that in such cases attendings need not prospectively justify their course of action to subordinates or colleagues. We noted that when their plans go awry there is no
everyday questioning such as they subject their housestaff to.
Such failures we coded as judgmental errors which we saw as a
privilege of rank. In the Mortality and Morbidity Conference
attendings pay for this privilege. They are obliged to explain how
eminences such as they made errors in judgment.[12] After the
subordinate's narration of the clinical history the attending steps
forward to field questions about the case. His taking over for the
subordinate indicates to his colleagues that the decisions in the
case were made by him and him alone, and that he alone will
answer for them. Difficult cases usually provoke a number of
questions from the audience, questions that are highly technical
in nature. For these cases, where a high degree of clinical uncertainty exists, the discussion reflects the academic and scientific
component of surgery. The conference becomes a seminar in
abstract problem solving. The longer the discussion continues,
the more complex it grows, the less subordinates participate, the
more discussion takes place among professional equals alone—
the attending surgeons. I shall hold off analyzing the attending's
account of the judgmental error until I have described the second
type of complex accounting situation since attending behavior is
similar in both of these situations.

The other complex failure an attending must explain is the
failure of a statistically preferred treatment, especially when the
consequences of that failure are grave. Here the surgeon must face
the personal consequences of the statistical concept of variance.
In the first complex accounting situation, the working consensus
of the group momentarily disintegrates. Individual opinions

predominate. There is no consensus as to what proper treatment is. In the second situation—the failure of a preferred treatment—the working consensus of the group is highlighted. Instead of procedure-oriented concerns and scientific detachment, we find patient-centered and emotionally colored statements. The patient's age and social status are often invoked. Attributions about the patient often reflect the surgeon's feelings. They speak of "this poor, unfortunate teenage boy," or "this courageous mother of five," or "this unpleasant, unattractive alcoholic." During these accounts there is often a macabre and irreverent humor in which the whole group shares compared to the sombre discussion when treatment alternatives are unclear:

> Roger, a chief resident, was accounting for his decision to remove the hemorrhoids of a patient in the end stages of cancer. The patient had not been able to withstand this normally routine procedure and had bled to death. The wisdom of operating on a patient in such a compromised position was questioned. Roger replied: "He was in great pain from the hemorrhoids—he really was. Everyday on rounds he would beg us to do something for it. We agreed, but only reluctantly. But I can tell you one thing: When he died, he sure as hell died without pain from hemorrhoids." It was some time before order was restored (Mortality and Morbidity Conference).

Finally, when preferred treatments fail, the audience often offers supportive remarks to the surgeon involved, such as "We all have a few cases like this," or "It's a mystery to me." In extreme cases the moderator of the conference will place an arm on the shoulder of the speaker before he returns to his seat. In these cases, attendings also accept and publicly acknowledge their responsibility by taking control of the proceedings from their subordinates. How they use this control to dramatize the distance between themselves and their subordinates and to legitimate their authority is the topic we now turn to.

In both complex accounting situations, the major ritual that substitutes for the public sanctioning of attendings occurs. Attending surgeons publicly abase themselves before an audience

of their colleagues and subordinates. They publicly claim that
they made mistakes in the handling of the case. They put on the
hair shirt, as the argot of surgery has it. When an attending puts
on the hair shirt, he points out to the group what lessons he
learned from treating the patient; he explains why he might better
have followed some other course of action; and he urges all to
consider the case before acting on similar cases in the future. The
hair shirts the attending dons in each of these two complex accounting situations are slightly different from one another. In the
first type of case, the attending points out what clinical evidence
he in retrospect seems to have valued too little, that is, why he
made his miscalculation and how he will correct it in the future.

In the discussion of the death of a sixty-eight-year-old woman
on the cardiac service, the attending in charge of the case
said the patient's death presented two questions to him:
(1) should the woman have been operated on in the first place,
and (2) should she have been taken off antibiotics. He then
claimed that the patient's death indicated that he was wrong
for deciding to operate in the first place. He then lectured
the group on the parameters one must evaluate in choosing
to operate or not (emphasizing as he did the parameter whose
importance he paid too little attention to). This finished,
he gave a similar lecture on the use of antibiotics (Mortality
and Morbidity Conference).

Two infant deaths were presented by the pediatric surgery
service. Both cardiac patients with similar problems were
presented at the same time. After the recital of the two
clinical histories, the attending in charge took over. He discussed the technical problems involved in handling the case
and what research needed to be done before one could hope
to successfully treat these patients. Then he claimed that
"as it stands now anybody that comes to me with this problem
already has their ticket punched"—a reference to the inevitability of death. He then gave a very short speech about how
both patients were very young infants and how these young
infants accounted for almost all the mortality among pediatric
cardiac patients. He claimed that such patients represented
the greatest challenge in the field and that he hoped the next

generation of surgeons would be able to solve these problems
and wonder how come his generation lost all these cases. His
presentation lasted six minutes and no questions were asked
(Mortality and Morbidity Conference).

With this hair shirt, the attending demonstrates for his subordinates the behavior that he expects when they make lesser
technical and judgmental errors. He shows how he has recon-
sidered his behavior as the emerging events brought them into
question and he shows what lessons such reconsiderations have
brought home to him.

The second type of hair shirt demonstrates a different type of
expected behavior from subordinates, that is, total integrity and
complete disclosure of shortcomings rather than any attempt at
cover-up. In the second type of case, when an attending puts on
the hair shirt he grounds the failure in his improper supervision of
his subordinates. Attendings believe that these are deaths and
complications that should just not occur and when such misadventures do occur, they blame themselves for their own lack of
foresight. While privately they damn their subordinates for what
they see as treacherous behavior for a physician, attendings
publicly state that it was their negligence and not that of their
housestaff that accounts for the failure:

After the case of Mr. Will was presented, Arthur sprang
from his chair and said that he had a few words to say in the
matter. He said: "I think that this case represents all the
things that are wrong with the hierarchy of a teaching hospital. Here we have one of society's unfortunates. Mr. Will
came to us with no kith or kin. He was comatose when he
arrived and we still really don't know who Mr. Will is or why
he came to us. The first in the comedy of errors made on
this man was made by the medical service. The decision by
them not to dilate his abdomen was tantamount to gross neglect. I only mention the medical service because they are
here and because I'm now going to turn to the errors we
made in treating this man. First, I made a fundamental error
this early in the training year in allowing the chief resident to operate solo in this emergency. We should have

learned from experience never to do this. In our defense we discussed this case with the resident involved over the phone. The third guilty party is the chief resident involved. By not calling for help when he ran into trouble, the resident took undue risk with the patient's life. Fortunately, the case looks like it will have a happy ending because of some heroic efforts made to undo the damage. Now, Mr. Will is an old, unattractive, abandoned, cirrhotic black man whom we almost abandoned to surgical pathology. Our surgical responsibility rests evenly with our unattractive as well as our more attractive patients. In this case, we have clearly committed surgical immorality." When he finished, no one spoke (Mortality and Morbidity Conference).

After the presentation of a case in which there had been a complication from the insertion of a subclavian catheter, Dr. Stone rose to speak: "This case is unfortunate and represents a want of supervision on my part. Clearly, this is a simple error in technique that could have been avoided if the resident had had proper instruction. The insertion of a subclavian catheter can be a very tricky business. It requires poise and confidence. It should be carefully supervised. Unfortunately, it is one of those procedures that we are least likely to monitor. All too often, we instruct our residents to insert subclavian catheters as we walk off the floor on our way home for the night. We should not—as I did in this case—do this. We should make sure our subordinates are properly equipped to do this and we should be there to provide help until we are confident our housestaff can do these things on their own. It is our responsibility to be available and provide instruction. We cannot always count on our housestaff to properly assess the trickiness of techniques" (Mortality and Morbidity Conference).

In the first type of account, the attending takes total responsibility for all decisions and for the way that they were carried out. He indicts his judgment in handling the case. In the second case, he takes responsibility for decisions, even maintains they were correct, but tries to separate himself from the way the decisions were carried out. He does not totally excuse his subordinates but blames himself for allowing their performance to proceed unchecked. If the subordinate makes a mistake it is only because his superordinate allowed him to do so. On the face of it, this is quite an admission for an attending to make; it is tantamount to the confession of a normative error. The attending tells all assembled that his commitment to patient care was wanting and some patient was caused unnecessary suffering. The only redeeming feature of this confession is that it sets a standard for full and open disclosure and complete intellectual integrity that houseofficers are expected to match. In either case, when an attending puts on a hair shirt he admits error, points out the lessons in it, and urges all to consider these before hasty action in the future. Attendings wear a hair shirt because a death or complication, especially when unexpected, is a pretty damning piece of evidence that forces them to consider alternatives. However, that they so willingly admit error and humble themselves before a group of colleagues and subordinates seems strange. How are we to account for this practice which seems to run against the grain of human nature, which usually conceals, minimizes, and denies error?

Two factors seem most noteworthy. First, as attendings often state, one purpose of the Mortality and Morbidity Conference is to instill professional "superegos" in junior staff. When an attending puts on the hair shirt, he makes the working of his own professional superego transparent. He shows what considerations should inhibit a too hasty impulse to act. Second, these public confessionals serve to mitigate the rigid hierarchical authority system of a surgical service. When he dons the hair shirt, the superordinate humbles himself before an audience of many subordinates over whom he has complete career control and whom he chews out daily. The conference is the only occasion when an attending is open to criticism. That this is self-criticism rather than the more acrimonious and harder to bear ill judgment of others is important but beside the point. These public ritualized admissions of fallibility contrast sharply with the everyday behavior of attending surgeons and serve to mitigate it somewhat.

This interpretation of the hair-shirt ritual is given greater plausibility when we consider additional aspects of the practice. The humbling effects are ordinarily softened, either by other attendings who indicate that they would have handled the case in the same way or who cite similar examples from their own clinical history or by pathologists who indicate that the patient was ravaged by disease and beyond repair. More interestingly, "wearing the hair shirt" is a prerogative of status. Although junior staff are forced to wear the garment in the informal setting of rounds (in fact, having thought through a death or complication, admitting responsibility, and pointing out the clinical lesson learned is one of the ways they establish that they are competent and trustworthy), they are not allowed to wear the hair shirt in the public conference. In these cases, the breach between expectation and outcome is not satisfied until the attending offers his exposition of events. Even though a subordinate may know the facts of a matter, he cannot authoritatively resolve the confusion these facts create.

The attending's refusal to let subordinates wear the hair shirt in public is an attempt by senior surgeons to illustrate to junior surgeons what the acceptable limits of a professional superego are. Attendings want subordinates to be mindful of the consequences of their action; however, they do not want them to be overly scrupulous. They do not want excessive thought—an overestimation of risk—to inhibit clinically indicated action. By refusing to allow subordinates to blame themselves for certain failures, attendings show that professional second-guessing properly ends where professional authority ends. In so doing, they once again underscore the status differences among their ranks. There is a very subtle give-and-take going on in the Mortality and Morbidity Conference. On the one hand, attendings encourage subordinates to question the grounds for their action; yet on the other, attendings try to limit that questioning so that it does not impair the quick judgments necessary in surgery.

There is yet another reason why "wearing the hair shirt" is a privilege of rank; it would be unseemly in a junior surgeon. If a junior surgeon claims he is mistaken often enough, we must take him seriously. At this point in his career, when competence is always an issue, weekly self-incriminations would ill serve the junior surgeon. Also, the hair shirt might prove too attractive for the subordinate. He might wish to wear it too often and therefore not be self-critical enough to see how his performance can be improved, or he may never learn to discriminate between those failures which he can and cannot control. An unrestrained *mea culpa, mea culpa* ill fits the heroic ideal of grace under pressure into which surgeons are socialized. Now, this is not so for the attending surgeon who stands at the top of his profession. He has a luminous professional biography and history—his credentials are unshakeable. The cases in which he assumes responsibility are marginally worthless in assessing his competence. These pale in comparison to his great achievements. In fact, for the super- ordinate, putting on the hair shirt only emphasizes the surgeon's charity, humanity, and the scope of his wisdom. It allows him to round out his professional self by adding to it the secondary qualities associated with the healer in our culture: humility, gentleness, wisdom, and a certain wry acceptance of the universe that allows him to accept the limits of human activity. It allows him to express guilt without being consumed by it. Such expres- sions of guilt might consume the subordinate who does not yet have the same mastery. It is difficult to adopt a long-run perspec- tive and be philosophical without the stock of experience that encourages such wisdom. By allowing actions that cause guilt to be openly confessed, putting on the hair shirt is a form of institu- tionalized self-protection for attendings. At the same time, it communicates to subordinates that no one is perfect; it models for them the proper expression of guilt and teaches them to accept that such accidents are an inevitable, unfortunate, and intractable fact of professional life:

> The conference is for the housestaff really. First, we go
> through the dialogue to point out verbally, schematically, and
> theatrically the issues involved. It is a teaching device first
> and foremost. Second, it shows by example honesty and lack
> of immunity from the problems of the profession. It teaches
> that these problems will be with them their whole professional
> life. Third it's good for our own characters to admit mistakes.

Deaths and complications are great levelers in surgery. It
teaches that you are not the archangel Gabriel, that you
bleed when cut (Attending).

Putting on the hair shirt is the major and most striking activity
of formalized retrospective peer review. By this practice surgeons
excuse their mistakes by admitting them. The major punishment
of the practice is the embarrassment of a public confessional and
the pain the outcome itself actually causes the surgeon's conscience. As a form of social control, this admission of error rests
on the self-surveillance and self-reports of the individuals involved. In this sense, it is part of a chivalrous code of behavior.
Moreover, when an individual can wear the hair shirt, he has
more or less passed beyond the few available social controls
surgery has. So this is a hair shirt on the outside only; for the
wearer it has the silken lining of unconditional professional support. Nevertheless, it is proper to ask how common it is for
attendings to avoid this public embarrassment and to conceal
their failure and what the consequences of this behavior are.

The actual extent of concealment is difficult, if not impossible,
to measure. On Able and Baker Services we never observed such
activity. Yet all subordinates are able to recall cases when services
they were on absented themselves from the conference at strategic
points. Both superordinates and subordinates take a dim view of
such behavior; and although all agree it occurs, they also agree its
actual extent is rare. When such behavior is even suggested it is
met with severe distaste:

Paul asked Mark if Carlos's wound infection was on this
week's Mortality and Morbidity agenda. Mark replied: "Of
course." A student asked: "Why did you do that? You
schedule the cases yourself. You know that there's no one
looking over your shoulder to check out what should be at
M&M." Mark answered sharply: "That would be no good. A
physician that doesn't own up to his own mistakes is no better
than the shit that's draining out of Carlos's wound. No, this
leak in the anastomosis is clearly a technical error. I still
don't know what caused it. It could have been caused by any
of a multitude of factors. But it is our error. No doubt about

it, and we're going to have to take our lumps for it" (Able Service).

Sure, a few complications are hidden by senior staff. I know of three right now. It's predictable behavior from the individuals involved. It's a case of insecurity leading to weakness and weakness leading to dishonesty. The individuals involved are destroyed by this. They lose all credibility and professional respect (Attending).

The refusal of superordinates to wear the hair shirt is a serious breach, comparable to the lack of total disclosure attendings demand from housestaff. Those attendings who do not wear the hair shirt often enough or who, worse yet, conceal their complications, undermine their own authority with colleagues and subordinates.[13] Wearing the hair shirt and scrupulously reporting all operative misadventures serves as evidence to subordinates that an attending applies to his own work the same standards he applies to theirs. It serves as evidence to colleagues that he respects the highest professional ideals and is ready to sacrifice face to protect them.[14] An attending that is publicly honest and open about his own shortcomings earns the right to be arbitrary, stubborn, and dogmatic on occasion because his own integrity and motives are beyond question. He has demonstrated that he is dedicated above all to the improvement of patient care.

five

Climbing the
Pyramid:
Professional
Control and
Moral Identity

So far our discussion of social control in a surgical training program is incomplete. We have analyzed how blameworthy failure is discovered and distinguished from blameless failure. We have seen what surveillance techniques attendings use to determine who guilty parties are and how guilty they are. We have analyzed the dramaturgic legitimation of the considerable authority that allows an attending to act as a houseofficer's defender and/or prosecutor at the same time that he is his judge. Yet so far this discussion neglects the enduring punishments superordinates impose on subordinates while emphasizing such obvious and immediate disciplinary tactics as verbal scorn, public ridicule, and icy and contemptuous avoidance. In this chapter I remedy this defect by extending our temporal perspective from the recurrent everyday level to the longer-run perspective of the fifteen-month period in which a cohort of subordinates is evaluated. As we move conceptually from the level of incident to the level of biography we shall see that attendings do more than get angry at erring houseofficers, they also exert a most powerful influence on an individual's career path. At the end of a subordinate cohort's first fifteen months of training, attendings decide which houseofficers will be allowed to complete their surgical training at Pacific, which will be forced to pursue careers at less elite institutions, and which will be advised to give up surgical careers altogether. Attending surgeons make these gatekeeping decisions at a faculty meeting of the Department of Surgery. This meeting—or meetings, if the decisions are particularly difficult to make—is the last time subordinates are judged formally as a group.[1] It is a nodal moment in a surgical career and it goes without saying that it warrants our careful consideration. In this chapter, we give a brief description of the context that surrounds the attending's decision making, show how attendings apply a "value-added" logic to evaluate houseofficers, and demonstrate that the promotion decision is a presumptive moral licensing that provisionally admits or blackballs a subordinate from the fraternity of academic surgeons.

The Context

The surgical training program at Pacific is a "pyramid" program. Each year more interns are accepted than there are places for senior residents. Part of this surplus is planned for. These are interns with a primary interest in one of the surgical specialties, such as orthopedics or urology, who must gain some experience in basic surgical techniques before they enter the subspecialties. The remainder of the interns are those who hope to advance to the top of the pyramid. In the year for which we made our observations, six people competed for four slots. The number of slots was, however, negotiable, and in fact only three positions were filled. The attendings at Pacific chose to operate with one empty slot rather than either accept one of their own subordinates whom they found wanting, or submit to the organizational humiliation of filling a position with an intern who had failed to climb the pyramid at some other elite institution. The fact that attendings were willing to fill only three positions despite funding for a fourth is very significant. It indicates how seriously they take their "gate-keeping" functions; attendings were not willing to compromise standards merely because the budget allowed it.

The decision to leave a position empty caused much debate. The attendings originally voted to fill four slots. Two factors were decisive: such staffing had been the tradition of the program, an expectation that subordinates had been laboring under for the last fifteen months and, more important, an increased case load was anticipated for the following year. There were many reasons for this expectation. First, there was a "maturing" of the faculty. There was a recent increase in the number of attendings at Pacific and these new attendings were building their practices quickly. Second, efforts were under way to make the referral of more difficult cases from community hospitals to Pacific more formal and more efficient. There was some resistance to these colonizing efforts by the community hospitals but it seemed clear to all attendings that much progress had been made. Legislation making programs for continuing medical education compulsory in such community hospitals served to strengthen the position of the attendings at Pacific and increase their optimism. However, after the attendings surveyed the second-year crop of subordinates and found it wanting and after they decided it was unwise to allow a member of the first-year group to skip a rank, the attendings reversed their original decision and filled only three positions. After reaching this decision, a number of attendings expressed some relief that the closing of the state-run facility to which they were committed to providing coverage offered a convenient "PR" reason for closing ranks unexpectedly. By this public or official reason, these attendings hoped to sidestep the unpleasantness that a direct confrontation with the real reason—a shortage of residents with acceptable skills—would have necessitated. Facing the real reason squarely was painful to attendings who may have had to revise cherished notions about their own and the department's preeminence in the field and painful to subordinates who may have had to revise notions about their own worth.

Since such a weighty matter was not easily resolved, analyzing the questions it raised tells us much about Pacific as an institution. The issues discussed by the attendings in resolving this staffing problem reveal many of their concerns as medical educators. The question of the very steepness of the pyramid itself was raised as a general concern. The attendings felt that too steep a pyramid would encourage an unhealthy competition which would undermine the teamwork necessary for a high level of care. All attendings recalled with horror past times when the pyramid had grown too steep and it was difficult to obtain cooperation among residents. On the other hand, the faculty feared that a too gently sloping pyramid discouraged one external incentive for high-quality performance. Proper staffing was a mechanism for encouraging and restraining competition. Next, there was the question of what number of residents was consistent with the

program's primary goal of training high-quality academic surgeons. With overstaffing at the senior levels, the danger exists that
each senior resident does not get his share of emergencies and
challenging cases and so is unprepared for all the contingencies
he must face when released from training. Moreover, if standards
were compromised to admit staff to senior ranks of training,
attendings complained that the effort necessary to make the less-
qualified competent is taken from the effort necessary to make
the more-qualified superior. Attendings were convinced that such
a trade-off was inconsistent with the training program's present
reputation and goals as well as its future pretensions. Also,
attendings questioned what number of senior residents was
proper to insure that each of them would have an intense enough
relationship with their apprentices to assure that he would have
an impact on a houseofficer's thinking and his career. Such a
consideration is very important to attendings for they feel that
those they train and brand with their personal stamp contribute
to their own personal reputation as well as the organization's.
Some attendings state that those they train are in the long run
more important than their research or clinical contributions:

> I was talking to Dr. Grant. It was late in the afternoon and we
> were alone in the doctor's lounge. He said: "Are you going
> tonight to hear Dr. Daily of Eastern Hospital speak? You really
> should, you know. You can learn a lot from seeing him. He is
> a very distinguished surgeon—one of the most creative sur-
> geons in America. You can learn a lot from seeing him. You
> know, he has never trained anyone of prominence. And in
> academic surgery that is what counts most—whom you have
> trained. Long after your research is forgotten and your papers
> are outdated, people will remember you by whom you have
> trained. And Daily has trained no one—at Eastern—where
> he gets the pick of the top talent. You know why? He can't
> work with residents. He has to compete with them. He has to
> dominate them. And he winds up crushing them. Go hear
> him talk. He can tell you a lot about surgery" (Baker Service).

The debate over how many positions to fill is, for attendings at
Pacific, a much more complex problem than arriving at the
proper solution to an equation balancing the demand for services

and the supply of servers. It is also a debate about what members see as the character of their institution and its proper mission. At Pacific attendings regulated the supply of servers mindful of, but not contingent on, the demand for services. Such a stance was one they felt was consistent with the training program's primary goal, producing surgeons capable of making both academic and clinical contributions. It is easy enough to imagine how other hospitals of a different order than Pacific may see staffing more narrowly as a supply-demand problem. For example, community hospitals whose primary mission is to provide service might determine the number of residents more with an eye to antici-pated case load and local market considerations than the at-tendings at Pacific, who can within limits regulate demand by refusing less interesting referrals and accepting only those minor cases necessary to fulfill the program's need to provide cases for the less experienced.

Despite the debate over how many positions to fill, when it got down to cases the decision to promote or not was made indepen-dent of the original understanding to fill four slots. So when it turned out that the attendings felt that they had only three qualified residents, they reversed their original decision to staff four positions. Had there been five qualified residents, then I feel that the attendings would have been reluctant to lose a good prospect. Before the discussion of individual cases, attendings reminded each other that the training program had a great deal of built-in flexibility and that should there be a surfeit of qual-ified residents in the group, they had a number of options. For example, a resident could be asked to step out of the queue and work on a laboratory project and then return to the program at a later date. Just as there was no need to accept the unqualified because of excessive demand, there was no reason to reject the qualified because of a temporary embarrassment of riches. On a whole, it seemed that the immediate needs of the organizational environment exerted less influence on the decision-making pro-cess than did longer-run commitments to professional excellence.

Given this commitment to professional excellence, how is it determined in any particular case whether an individual is

qualified or not? Attendings evaluate the performance of subordinates in written recommendations. These letters are entered
in a subordinate's personnel file and are the official record of
his performance. In the fifteen-month period before decision
making, a subordinate will rotate through between eight and
twelve services. Each of these services is run by two or three
attendings. So, for the time period involved, subordinates ac-
cumulate approximately twenty-four letters of recommendation.
These letters range in length from a simple letter grade to a few
words to a few paragraphs. They also vary considerably in
specificity. Only one resident evaluation of the over 100 we
perused mentioned a specific incident critical or supportive of
a resident's performance. More commonly, letters will speak in
generalities. They will state that a resident has "some difficulty
getting along with staff or other residents," or that "there is fairly
common friction between this resident and nurses," or that "he is
still occasionally bothered by personality conflicts with his co-
workers," and not mention what these difficulties are. Letters of
praise are likewise very vague, often stating nothing more about a
resident than that "he is outstanding in every respect," or that
"he should have a very promising career."

These evaluations of resident performance are interesting
documents in their own right. They indicate how very consequential typifications are made and supported by only the merest
shards of evidence. These evaluations illustrate the various
interpretive procedures by which performance and performers
are labeled. There is labeling by analogy, that is, statements of
the type that "at this stage in his training, X reminds me of Y"
(where Y is an old resident). There is labeling by hypothesis, that
is, statements of the type, "I expect a person like X to perform in
such and such a fashion if confronted by situation Y." There is
labeling by negative or positive hyperbole, that is, statements of
the type that "this resident is so bad or good that words cannot
describe his performance." There is labeling by elliptical allusion, that is, statements of the type that allude to a specific
problem that a subordinate has without ever providing an
example. All these techniques indicate that labeling does not

proceed through a careful sifting and documentation of cases, but through artfully employed rhetorical devices. One reason that careful documentation is unnecessary is the respect that attendings have for each other's clinical wisdom. The rhetorical devices of analogy, hypothesis, hyperbole, and allusion are a shorthand language that all colleagues understand, share, and employ to describe what are very complex judgments of performance. The nature of the evaluations is itself prima facie evidence of the importance of clinical judgment and the attendings' claims to it. Were this not so, efforts would be made to make the evaluations more standardized, rendering them more comparable and replicable, that is, scientific.

Be that as it may, these evaluations are, for our purposes, not very useful. They show us what kinds of facts about houseofficers attendings find worthy of recording. They show us how everyday experience is generalized. But the documents in and of themselves tell us little about the decision-making process of promotion. To understand this, we have to look to the dynamics of the promotion meeting itself. We have to analyze the decision making and not the documents that are invoked as a background resource to justify a particular decision.

Value-Added Logic and Sorting

At the promotion meeting when attendings evaluate each resident's performance, they have three options before them: (1) they can decide that no amount of training will ever make a resident a competent surgeon and recommend that he try another speciality; (2) they can decide that, while a resident will in all likelihood become a competent surgeon, he lacks the wherewithal to serve in an elite atmosphere, and recommend that he try another training program; (3) or they can decide that a resident is competent and admit him to the ranks of senior residency. The attending problem is to sift through the available talent and sort it. Superordinates discipline subordinates in the long run by excluding them from their professional networks and they reward them by including them. The main mechanism of social control is sorting.[2]

Sorting as a process involves ordering what would otherwise be a chaotic congregation of elements by categories and then within categories, subcategories. As a process, sorting operates within a value-added logic (Smelser 1962), that is, the result of each sort narrows the range of possible outcomes for the next sort. In evaluating residents and thus setting their career options, attendings apply such a value-added logic. This logic is appropriate to their task at hand—putting each subordinate in his proper place.[3] As the work of Bittner (1967) on police discretion and Cicourel (1969) on juvenile justice show, sorting is a standard operating procedure for social control agents. Sorting is applied typification. Moreover, value-added sorting is a basic socially structured cognitive process which we all use to order, name, and thereby behave appropriately in social situations. Our task here is not to account for the basic process, but to show how attendings employ it to rank subordinates and exercise professional control.

The first sorting question is, Does an individual possess the technical capacity to be a surgeon? Two of the six individuals in the cohort I observed were judged as lacking the motor skills and the temperament necessary for surgery. Such determinations were arrived at quickly:

> "The next person on our list is Smith," said Dr. Gray, the department chairman. Dr. White comments: "He was a mistake. I think we should advise him to take a career in something other than surgery. I'm surprised he's on this list. I thought I had convinced him six or seven months ago to go into another specialty." Dr. Peters: "He's an absolute clunker. He has no promise." Dr. Pines: "He should be in another specialty." Dr. Ross: "There is absolutely no hope of training him to be a competent surgeon." Then Dr. Gray says, "Okay. Then we are all agreed. I'll talk to Smith and see if we can work something out for him. Perhaps in one of the other departments here" (Department Meeting).

The faculty were agreed that Smith lacked the requisite skills necessary to be a surgeon at any institution, but despite this, they

were not willing to banish him from the ranks of the elite
altogether. What happened in his case was on each service that he
rotated through he made technical errors and failed to improve
over time. This was evidence for all that he could never be a
surgeon. However, on each service, Smith handled these errors in
a proper fashion. He recognized them quickly, reported them,
and made certain they were corrected. His repeated misadventures convinced his superordinates he lacked talent as a
surgeon. Nevertheless, his normative propriety convinced his
superordinates that, although Smith was in the wrong field, he
might be in the right place. They were ready to counsel him and
recommend him to colleagues in other departments at Pacific. The
attendings viewed Smith as a simple tracking problem: he had the
intelligence and integrity necessary to be a member of the medical
elite and attendings concerned for his welfare wanted to see him
placed properly. Their willingness to help Smith was encouraged
by Smith's growing sense that he had made an error in choosing a
surgical career, by his willingness to discuss this openly with
attendings, and by his eagerness to work out more viable options.

The faculty agreed as quickly as they did in Smith's case that a
second candidate, Jones, lacked the technical skills necessary for
a surgical career. But in this second case, they had grave doubts
about whether Jones had any place in the medical profession at
all. Jones had combined technical maladroitness with an inability
to admit mistakes and difficulties in communicating with patients and staff. This had led on occasion to small correctable
errors growing into catastrophes.

> Dr. Gray opened discussion of Jones by reporting: "Jones has
> had a lot of problems over the last fifteen months. This
> morning, I talked with him and told him that an inability
> to communicate with peers and patients was not a quality we
> were looking for in our residents. I suggested to him that he
> meet with Dr. Cantor in psychiatry to discuss whatever
> personal problems he has before he makes any plans to con-
> tinue his career in any capacity. He was quite adamant that
> he needed no help and that he wanted to be a surgeon."
> Dr. Grant said: "I did not know what to make of Dr. Jones

his first few days on our service, but I have reluctantly come to
the conclusion that this man is sick. I don't trust him around
my patients." An attending asked, "How do you mean sick—
physically or mentally?" Dr. Arthur answered, "Mentally. He's
off his rocker. Totally out to lunch. He needs help and he
needs it quick. The question is not whether we should keep
him, but whether he should finish out the year. In my mind, I
wonder if he's on drugs." Dr. Gray then said: "As I said before
when I gave him the option of seeing Dr. Cantor, he was totally
opposed to it." Dr. Grant added: "There is no doubt he needs
help. Yesterday in clinic he was really around the bend. He
couldn't focus on patients. You could not have a conversation
with him. He couldn't deal with anything." Dr. Peters commented that "it doesn't sound like much has changed over the
course of a year. Maybe he has a brain tumor." Dr. Ross said:
"If he has a problem, I don't think we could in good conscience
let him go without offering him help. I think we have a
responsibility to see that he gets proper care. But our responsibility to our patients comes first. If there is doubt about his
stability, we cannot continue to let him see patients." Dr. Gray
then summarized the comments about Jones by saying: "Then
we are agreed. Not only will Jones not be offered a position,
but he will not be allowed to return to duty until he is investi-
gated by someone in neuropsychiatry" (Meeting).

The attendings felt some responsibility for Jones as a person
under their care. However, Jones' breaches were so consistent and
so consistently denied by Jones that immediate expulsion was
necessary. Unlike Smith, Jones was not a tracking problem. He
was a total problem that attendings wished to rid themselves of
entirely by shifting responsibility to the psychiatry department.

The contrast between the handling of Smith and Jones supports my argument about the differences between technical and
normative error and also suggests inherent limits to professional
control. A lack of requisite technical skill disqualifies one for a
surgical career but not for a career as a physician. If one has made
a mistake in choosing to be a surgeon, and if that mistake is
compounded by acceptance in a surgical training program, it can
be corrected. The cost of the mistake is the time the subordinate

spent in training and the effort superordinates wasted trying to teach him. However, as long as the subordinate complies with the norms of his role, the cost to patients is kept at a minimum. Moreover, while the subordinate's performance demonstrates to his superordinates that he will never be a surgeon, at the same time it convinces them that in the proper field he has a contribution to make. The problem is wedding aptitudes and inclinations to the proper clinical area. On the other hand, an absence of technical and normative skills indicates to superordinates that an individual is unfit to be a physician. Unfortunately, such knowledge comes too late. The subordinate has already graduated from medical school. He is a doctor. Superordinates as agents of professional control can block some career options. They can suggest that an individual get help. But they cannot block all career options. Nor can they force an individual to seek help. Their jurisdiction is limited. If they are willing to take enough trouble, they can perhaps block training in many institutions. But there are internships that go abegging every year; and, ironically, failing at Pacific may recommend an individual to a more lackluster organization. A sufficiently stubborn individual can get trained and eventually licensed to practice medicine, even if he has to give up his ambition to be a board-certified surgeon. Attendings know that there is nothing that they can do to stop this. They realize the market for medical school graduates is highly differentiated. In some sectors, it is a buyer's market; in others, it is a seller's. This split-market structure does much to frustrate attendings' efforts at control.

The four remaining candidates passed the first "sort," that is, it was agreed by all attendings that these residents possessed the technical skills necessary for careers as surgeons. The second sorting question concerns a person's "teachability," that is, his ability to learn from his mistakes and improve on his performance. Attendings ask, Will this person mature? They use three indicators for this: a resident's relations with patients and nurses, his general level of enthusiasm, and his relationship to and with attending authority. Of the four residents who passed the first sort, three passed the second. There was little disagree-

ment about the three candidates that passed the second sort;
consensus was quickly reached. On the other hand, much
controversy surrounded the fourth candidate. He was debated
over one hour at the first promotion meeting. The attendings
were not able to come to any decision regarding his future, and
scheduled a second meeting to continue discussion. Discussion at
the second meeting lasted over two hours. At the end of this
meeting, the attendings declined to offer the resident a position.
Before discussing this long debate, it is helpful to look at the
decision to retain the other three residents. This will provide us a
useful contrast.

Consensus to keep the three qualified residents was quickly
arrived at. No attending mentioned any problem that arose and
recurred with any of the three residents. Discussion started with a
statement of praise for the resident. This was echoed by an
attending from a second service and then from a third. After the
third attending spoke, others nodded their agreement. Gray,
seeing that his colleagues were of one mind, then announced:
"Okay, we're agreed. We'll keep him." In the first promotion
meeting, which lasted three hours, only fifteen minutes, more or
less, were spent discussing all three promoted residents. A typical
exchange went as follows:

> Dr. Gray: "Okay, Thomas is next." Dr. Arthur: "Top-drawer.
> He's very quiet, but also very resourceful with patients, who
> like him a lot." Dr. Peters: "Yes, we were quite pleased with
> his work on our service. He works hard and he's very con-
> scientious." Dr. Ross: "His growth has been very good. He
> reminds me of Stone at a similar stage in his career, and as his
> confidence grows he may—like Stone—become less quiet."
> Dr. Gray, summarizing: "This boy is a real sleeper. I get the
> impression from looking over his folder that our opinion of
> him has grown with each rotation. We're agreed to keep him"
> (Meeting).

Residents are accepted to Pacific with high expectations for
their performance based on their stellar records as medical
students. For the three residents promoted to the senior ranks,
these positive expectations were satisfied. The performance of

these residents serves as testimony to the wisdom of accepting them in the first place. Nothing much really needs to be said about them.

This is not so for the resident who on occasion displays great technical prowess combined with normative lapses. Attendings have difficulty in accounting for his failure to meet expectations, and difficulty in deciding what to do with him. Of this resident attendings are forced to ask, Can we make him change, and does his promise justify the high cost in terms of time and energy necessary to work this change? This is a difficult decision to arrive at for a number of reasons. Chief among these is the fact that attendings recognize that it is the very qualities which cause one to be vexed with and disappointed in subordinates that may allow one to be a creative and outstanding member of the medical elite. Brashness, aggressiveness, and even stubbornness are qualities that can make a subordinate insufferable and lead him to make normative errors, but they can also lead to discovery and high-quality care. Second, attendings are well aware that a number of luminous names in academic surgery washed out of their original training programs. In the case of the technically gifted, attendings wish to minimize the type 2 error, that is, dismissing a subordinate as unfit when he is extremely talented. They wish to minimize type 2 errors because they can become a public embarrassment to the department and the judgment of its members, and because qualified trainees who move on to different institutions are important for recruiting future trainees to the program. Third, there is the very real frustration for attendings of seeing a person of talent not fulfilling his potential, despite their best efforts to change this.

In this cohort, resident Josh Carter (whose difficulties with Dr. Arthur were detailed in chapter 2) posed the most difficult promotional problem for attendings. All were agreed on his talent and intelligence. At the same time, all agreed that Carter's work oscillated between the excellent and the lackluster:

Dr. Pines commented: "I agree with Fred in almost everything he says. This guy is talented and likable. There's no question about it. But I had to jump all up and down on him this spring to get him to do the work. If he operates, fine, he does a good job managing and observing the patient. But if he's not operating ... [doesn't finish the sentence, just shrugs his shoulders]." Then Dr. Arthur said: "My complaint is that he is unreliable unless he's doing the operating. When you call at night and ask Carter how things are and he says all right, what he means is that the patient he's scheduled to operate on won't die by morning. He doesn't know how the rest of the patients are doing" (Meeting).

The question that attendings had about Carter was, Was his unreliability a part of his character resistant to change, or was it rather a temporary condition caused by his not yet learning the humility appropriate to his station? Carter's experience both in medical school and at Pacific made it difficult to tell which was the case. Attendings reported times when their attempts to discipline Carter were immediately undone by other attendings, who extravagantly praised his work. This process in fact had its concomitant in the promotional meeting as negative statements about Carter were neutralized by positive ones:

Dr. Arthur: "He's great when he's interested. But if he's not, he doesn't give you or the patient the time of day." Dr. White: "I don't know about that, Bill. He worked hard for me and Ollie in September, which was our busiest time. He really stayed on top of things and really pulled a few chestnuts out of the fire." Another attending added: "Look, as I listen I can't escape the feeling that we all know surgeons like this. It seems to be a character type. The question is, do we want to be responsible for training that kind of person? This fellow never rotated through my service, so I don't know him, and I still can't tell from the discussion whether he has a character disorder or whether these problems will go away with maturity" (Meeting).

As the discussion of Carter continued, the attendings' ambivalence about him seemed to grow. He was credited with great talent, intelligence, and the ability to work long and hard hours when motivated to do so. He was damned with being on occasion unreliable, untrustworthy, slovenly, and churlish. Carter's failures, on the whole, were breaches of the standard decorum for care—he violated the rule of "no surprises" too often for attendings to ignore. These breaches of Carter did not always harm patients, but they were seen by attendings as more serious than failures which harmed patients but were rule-governed in terms of medical etiquette. Carter's skills and his shortcomings were so balanced that attendings were unable to come to any sort of decision about his future at the end of the first meeting. They decided to discuss Carter again in their next meeting in a month. The attendings decided to let him know that his future was not yet decided. They hoped that his reaction would give them a clue as to whether he was teachable, or an incorrigible.

In the four weeks that intervened between the first and second meeting, Carter gathered information about what happened at the attendings' meeting. He responded by sending emissaries to those attendings he felt most strongly opposed his retention, and by having extra letters of recommendation entered into his file. These responses angered the attendings and convinced them that Carter's problems were beyond their ability to treat. By mounting what one of his strongest supporters among attendings called a "lousy PR campaign," Carter had missed the point of his critics and proved himself incorrigible. He had shown himself so inattentive to the cues of others that he proved himself unteachable. Further, his response served as evidence that what his harshest critics claimed were his problems—a lack of integrity and a desire to take the easy way out—were true:

> Dr. Arthur said of Carter: "He lacks integrity. What he's done now shows it, and his work with us showed it. To give you an example, one day I asked him if something had been done, and he said it was taken care of. But when I got to the first floor, I found that it hadn't been done. So I asked him what had happened between the sixth floor and the first floor. He answered, 'Well, I gave the nurses orders.' He was probably innocent in the legal sense of the term, but he was guilty of being less than candid. I shudder to think of him as a chief resident." Dr. White said: "As you know, I defended him last month. But the way I feel right now, I don't think he has the maturity to be a chief resident" (Meeting).

After two hours, the attendings convinced themselves that Carter could be made into a competent surgeon but that they were not going to be the ones to take the trouble to do it. Dismissing Carter now, they decided, would serve all their interests best. Another position for him somewhere else could easily be arranged, and he would not be unduly stigmatized for his failure. On the attendings' part, they would be rid of a problem and have more time time for teaching that promised greater returns for their efforts. At the same time, by arranging Carter's placement elsewhere, the attendings at Pacific could continue to monitor his progress and welcome him back into their ranks should he begin to live up to his potential.

There is an irony in Carter's banishment from the medical elite. He was excluded for his inability to meet the expectations superordinates had for trustworthy subordinates. He had failed to properly internalize the norms of the doctor role while displaying great technical talent. Demoting Carter to a training program where the attendings were less professionally imposing than those of Pacific made it even less likely that Carter would accept superordinate authority and hence less likely he would internalize these norms. In addition, it was likely that his considerable technical talents would not develop to their fullest because of restricted clinical exposure. The attendings hoped that, all else having failed, Carter would learn a lesson from his exile from the elite. Given the available options, the punishment fit the crime; however, it was the one most likely to perpetuate it.

Although we have analyzed a cohort of only six, a small sample to be sure, the decisions of the promotion meeting feed back on and lend credibility to the observations of chapters 2, 3, and 4. First, technical and judgmental error is acceptable as long as it can be interpreted as an occasion for learning. However, when made too frequently, such errors discredit a subordinate as a potential surgeon. The commission and concealment of such errors discredit a subordinate as a potential physician entirely. However, the superordinate's ability to control the subordinate are limited. A morally discredited individual in one setting can still obtain license in another. Second, given that subordinates meet technical standards, normative ones become paramount. Those who meet them are embraced; those who do not are rejected. For those who have it, technical proficiency is a rather indifferent indicator of success. Normative compliance with superordinate expectations accounts for who will be retained or fired.[4] Even for those who lack technical proficiency, normative skills determine available alternatives. Attendings themselves are often required to demonstrate that they possess the qualities they demand of subordinates. Their intellectual integrity is displayed in the "hair-shirt" ritual, which models for subordinates the proper way to account for failure.

On Joining the Ranks

Attendings say of the subordinates that they accept into the ranks that "he's our kind of person," or "he's our people." Both phrases end discussion of a subordinate admitted to the ranks of the senior residency. Both phrases serve as a benediction to mark the passage of a subordinate from one whose trustworthiness and skill are always open to question to one who is accepted as a group member.

Besides securing his career for the moment, being certified as their kind of person by attendings has great meaning in the everyday life of the subordinate. When attendings claim that a person is their kind of person, this serves as a preliminary and presumptive moral licensing of that person. This moral licensing has a number of interactional concomitants. Chief among these is a more collegial and respectful treatment of the subordinate by attendings. Once promoted, subordinates are less often the target of attendings' anger and they are less likely to be seen as the responsible agents for culpable failure; as a consequence, they are less likely to be morally discredited.

In the third year of training, the subordinate who makes it that far is relieved of many of the cross-cutting pressures of his role which we saw as responsible for normative and quasi-normative error. The organization of ward work is left to those in the first two years of training. The senior resident is compelled to spend less time at the hospital either performing menial tasks or on call (although his total work hours are still somewhat staggering). He himself becomes dependent on those below him adhering to the rule of "no surprises." When this rule is not followed, the resident joins with the attending in trying to find out why and prevent its recurrence. However, if problems recur, the senior resident can find his attending's approval quickly withdrawn and find himself blamed for not exercising a tight enough control. But as a rule the senior resident is more a junior partner than a servant of the attending.

There are also other subtle changes that occur once one is admitted into the ranks. The third-year resident begins to call the younger attendings by their first names. His relations with older attendings are likely to become cordial, with much more mutual kidding. The third-year resident begins to do more teaching during rounds and ward work. He is allowed to enjoy more of the privileges of rank, and made to suffer less the burdens of initiation.

Admission into senior ranks provisionally admits one to a colleague network. One is seen as a member of the group that has passed the harshest of the initiation rites the profession has to offer. Attendings express this when they say they can "sleep well" knowing a particular resident is in charge. The first two years of training, subordinates are severely tested. For the last three years, they slowly gain acceptance as colleagues.

six

Conclusion

Failure to perform competently as a professional means two different things. First, there is failure to apply correctly the body of theoretic knowledge on which professional action rests. Failures of this sort are errors in techniques. For surgeons, we have identified two varieties of this type of error—technical and judgmental. Second, there is failure to follow the code of conduct on which professional action rests. Failures of this sort are moral in nature. Again for surgeons we have identified two varieties of moral failure—normative and quasi-normative. Moral failure is more often the subject of serious social control efforts than errors in techniques. This is to say, social control of the profession subordinates technical performance to moral performance. In conclusion, we shall examine this finding.

First, I shall examine the technical-moral distinction itself to see why moral breaches are considered more serious than technical ones. Then I shall relate type of error to its conspicuousness and to the response it evokes. I shall demonstrate that moral errors are more conspicuous than technical ones and that they arouse a stronger response. A discussion of these relationships informs us how professionals interpret their charter, tells us what license and mandate mean to the professional, and informs us what professionals mean when they claim to exercise professional self-control.

Technical vs. Moral Errors

Embedded in this ethnographic account is the contrast between technical errors, on the one hand, and moral errors, on the other.

Throughout we have seen that moral errors are more harshly treated. At the recurrent everyday level, technical errors are the occasion for restitutive sanctions while moral errors are an occasion for repressive ones. Superiors "support" those that make technical errors and "degrade" those who make moral ones. At the career level those who make technical errors are allowed to remain in the medical elite although they may not become surgeons, while those who make moral errors are banished from elite ranks although they are allowed to become surgeons elsewhere. Why is it that techniques are subordinated to morals? This is not a finding that the literature on professions with its emphasis on increasing specialization and cognitive rationality prepares us for. If anything, as the profession of medicine becomes more scientific, specialized, and bureaucratized, we would expect the opposite. As far as control of performance is concerned, we would expect impersonal evaluations of techniques to have priority over personal judgments of an individual's moral performance. How are we to account for the fact that the opposite is the case?

The explanation lies in the nature of the professional-client relationship. The professional agrees to apply his expertise to the client's problem in a manner that takes care not to abuse and/or exploit the client's helplessness. The professional agrees to protect the client's best interests. The physician does not promise to cure. The lawyer does not promise to win the case. The most that either can promise is to help as best he can and in a fashion consistent with the highest standards of the community. Now, in most professional-client relationships, the client has a great deal at stake. In fact, so much hangs in the balance that suspicion of the professional's motives and the appropriateness of his conduct is always a possibility. To defend against this, the professional proves how secondary his personal considerations are by placing himself in his client's service. He is available when the occasion demands. Moreover, professionals work to cultivate the impression that the only case they have of interest is the one before them now—the client being served at the moment.[1] A professional's claim that he will not benefit from the client's compromised position is backed by the sacrifices of time and energy that he makes for his client. In making these sacrifices, he matches what his client has at stake by a considerable investment of his own.

When things go awry, when the professional's efforts to aid his client fail whatever the reason, the professional's last line of defense—should he doubt himself, should his colleagues question him, should his clients or their representatives accuse him—is that he did everything possible. "Doing everything possible" is a moral defense and not a technical one. The individual claims his conduct is beyond question—that he did everything any other member of his profession might have done in similar circumstances—and that failure is accidental, incidental, and random. He claims that the case deviates so far from the average that it should be discarded from any sample of his normal performance. He argues that its inclusion so skews the sample of his normal work that one might be led to make unwarrantable inferences about his professional worth. The claim that he "did everything possible" is basically a claim to ethical conduct. When he claims that he did everything possible, the professional claims that he acted in good faith. Although results are open to debate, his conduct is not.

The challenges of "good faith behavior" come from three different sources, each at a different level of social organization. First, an individual can doubt himself. Here the claim of "good faith behavior" acts as an individual defense. The individual who convinces himself that he met all the obligations of his office assuages a guilty conscience. Second, a group of colleagues may question an individual's results. This is the professional group exercising its license and mandate. The group standard for what comprises "everything possible" may be stricter or harsher than an individual's. At Pacific the group standard demands sacrifices and imposes on the individual the obligation to recognize problems beyond his level of skill and to route these problems to the proper expert. These last two obligations are meant to assure the widest dispersal of high-quality care. Personal pride or self-interest then does not interfere with the ability to act in a client's interest. The ideal network of professionals is one in which each member in turn is expected to defer to his more knowledgeable colleague in order that skills and problems are properly and speedily aligned. Therefore, the moral behavior of doing everything possible is a guarantee of high-quality technical care. The third challenge of "good faith behavior" comes from outside the profession. Its formal expression is in the legal system. The rules of evidence for what constitutes good faith behavior are established by law rather than being part of an unwritten code. Here we confine ourselves to the professional code in general and to challenges of professionals in the organization specifically. We are concerned with the relation of the group to those members whose action is questioned.

The professional's last line of defense is a moral one because it is proper moral performance alone that substantiates a claim to proper technical performance when events mock such a claim. It is not the patient dying but the patient dying when the doctor on call fails to answer his pages that makes it impossible to sustain a case of acting in the client's interest. It is not losing the suit but losing the suit when representing a defendant while having substantial holdings in the plaintiff's company that mocks a claim of impartial justice. Moral error breaches a professional's contract with his client. He has not acted in good faith. He has done less than he should have. Such conduct is not honest and defensible but undercuts all the presumptions on which the professional-client relationship is based. For this reason moral errors are treated more seriously than technical ones. They undercut the very fabric of client-professional and professional-professional relationships. Hence the control of technical performance is subordinated to the control of moral performance; without the overarching moral system, the technical system is not amenable to control.

Two observations suffice to show the precedence of morals over techniques. First, the claims to excellence made by superordinates at Pacific are based not only on a technical superiority but also a moral superiority. They speak of "sweating blood" for patients or "really busting their butts on this one." The hours they work are a source of complaint but also a source of pride. Attendings feel it is their willingness to do more than their less luminous colleagues which distinguishes them more than anything else. It is this pride in working harder and doing more than others rather than a pride in the advanced medical technology available to them which informs their characterization of Pacific being a better hospital than others. Second, there is the following curious fact. The statistical limit which separates acceptable from unacceptable technical performance has never been firmly established. We do not know how many wound infections make a surgeon incompetent, nor do we know how much undiseased tissue he must remove before his honesty is thrown into question. Here professional standards are not established. Yet the minimum number of moral breaches needed to dismiss a professional from practice is clear-cut: one will do. One breach of professional ethics is all that is necessary to expel a physician from a hospital's staff or disbar a lawyer. In practice, of course, it is rare that a single infraction is so severe as to warrant this response.

The argument should not be pushed too far. We are not claiming that technical performance is unimportant. We are saying that normative, that is, moral, standards are the organizing principle of a professional community. It is worth noting that technical and moral performances are poles of a continuum. In some professions the continuum is quite truncated and any technical error is also a moral one: air-traffic controllers are a good example. In other professions, the continuum is quite long, so long that "not busting your butt" and not doing everything possible—restraining rescuer impulses—can be interpreted as part of proper therapy: psychiatry is a good example. The fact that this is the case allows professionals to accept the occasional technical error even when its consequences for the patient may be grave; defends them psychologically, socially, and legally against charges of exploiting a client's helplessness; and assures the client that his best interests are cared for.

Conspicuous
Performances

The above proof is a rather slender peg on which to hang an argument. We need to demonstrate that the technical control of performance is subordinated to moral controls with stronger data than any we have put forth. In the introduction I claimed that one good reason for studying surgeons in order to investigate social control processes was that their performances were inherently more conspicuous than those of physicians in other specialties. Simply stated, what a surgeon does is more obvious than what a psychiatrist does. We accept as a commonsense assumption that for performance to be labeled "deviant," it has to be somehow observable. Of all medical performances, surgical ones are most observable. After all, it is only these performances that are said to take place in a theater. If our contention is correct that in the concern for social control there is subordination of technical performances to moral ones, we would expect the control of techniques to be a less conspicuous part of the environment than control of morals.

This is, in fact, what we found. Surgeons are loath to judge the technical performance of others. Surgeons routinely condemn results without condemning the performance. They claim that "unless they were there they do not know what kind of situation the surgeon faced, what kinds of factors may have compromised his ability to perform the optimal procedure." They add that "they cannot say for certain what they would have done in the same situation." Because of the multitude of factors that influence judgment and confound results, the social control of techniques remains inconspicuous. When and where it occurs, such control is built into the fabric of everyday life as minidiscussions of surgical problems, as anecdotes or horror stories, as hypothetical questions for future considerations, or as mild rebukes. Individuals are not separated from the work group nor is action seen as in any way "nonnormal" by members of the surgical service.

The fact that controls of techniques are not a conspicuous

feature of group life underscores the problematic and probabilistic nature of medical practice, what Fox (1957*a*) identifies as the theme of uncertainty in medicine. There are three sources of uncertainty. There are inherent limits to medical knowledge itself; there is the inability of any one physician to master the entire corpus of available knowledge; and there is the difficulty in deciding in any particular case between the limits of the science and the limits of the person. When failure is technical, its source lies in one or some combination of these three sources of uncertainty. To cope with his own uncertainty and to suspend judgment about the failure of others is something practitioners learn early in a medical career. In an unpublished paper on the autopsy as a rite of passage, Fox (1957*b*) points out that prosectors are careful to specify, in cases where premortem diagnoses do not accord with postmortem findings, the good clinical evidence which informs incorrect diagnosis and treatment. Pathologists are careful not to impugn the motives, skills, or intelligence of the clinician involved.

The point here is that one learns that such a thing as honest errors exist and that all physicians make them. These things happen. There are generally good reasons that one can suggest post hoc for them. It is therefore not proper to damn such results with hindsight. When physicians act in "good faith," the reasons for failure are routinely recoverable and excusable. Moreover, it is assumed that the physician acting in good faith will learn from his failures. There is a general reluctance to let a technical failure be a conspicuous occasion for social control since its sources are so variegated, since the decisions demanded are so subtle and complex, since it happens to everyone, and since it is believed that the responsible physician will draw the proper lessons from the evidence.

While the social control of technical performance is inconspicuous, the control of moral performance is a very conspicuous feature of the environment. With errors of technique, it is never completely clear whether the fault lies in the individual or in the field. However, when the error is a moral one—a case of being improperly oriented to tasks at hand—an individual's liability is quite clear. The social control of moral performance is quite conspicuous. Dedication, hard work, and a proper reverence for role obligations are all readily apparent. A want of interest or enthusiasm in a subordinate is quickly noticed by a superior. From this evidence, superordinates are quick to infer that an underling has serious problems that will interfere with his becoming a high-quality physician. The subordinate's good faith is put into question by his behavior. The judgments that are suspended for errors in technique are not suspended here.

There are three senses in which moral performance and its control are more conspicuous than technical performance and its control. First, subordinates are constantly revealing their moral worth to superiors in a variety of manners: by their degree of attentiveness as they hold retractors,[2] by their affect as they discuss clinical problems, by their rapport with patients, and by their resourcefulness in getting things done. Superiors take all these as indicators of a person's moral performance. Differences in moral performance among subordinates are often greater than differences in technical performance, especially given the restrictions of a strictly regulated division of labor. Moral performance is more conspicuous than technical performance to begin with because superiors find it easier to read a subordinate's moral performance than his technical performance. Deficiencies in moral performance say more about an individual's capacity to improve and become a reliable colleague than do deficiencies in technical performance, which may speak to momentary and easily correctable shortcomings.

The heightened meaningfulness of moral performance over technical performance leads to a second way in which moral performance is highly conspicuous as a basis of social control: namely, moral performance seems more consequential in career-tracking decisions than technical skill. Letters of recommendation or condemnation cite moral character more commonly than mastery of the body of knowledge on which the profession rests.

Despite being talked to several times by Dr. Grant and myself, this man has a tendency to regard the patient as just

so much operative experience, and if he is not doing the
"cutting and sewing," he is just not interested. He avoids the
operating room when he is not going to be the operating
surgeon, and takes little interest in cases that he does not find
appealing or challenging. In short, he has not performed with
the maturity and dependability that one expects of a resident
of his maturity in years and apparently this is merely a contin-
uation of past problems.... At this juncture, I just cannot
visualize him as a chief resident in surgery as I would be
afraid of his slipshod methods and his cavalier attitudes
toward responsibility and toward his patients
(Department of Surgery).

Letters of praise routinely cite an individual's flexibility, dependability, and sensibility. When asked what they look for in
housestaff, attendings cite what they call the three A's: "avail-
ability, affability, and ability—in that order." At the promotion
meeting, the cutting edge in problematic cases was a person's
moral performance. Moral performance governs the sorting of
trainees into professional networks. There is a double irony in the
fact that technical performance is less conspicuous than moral
performance as a basis of social control. One would, of course,
assume that moral worth is more difficult to infer from behavior
than technical worth rather than vice versa. Is it not believed that,
after all, character resides in a more hidden recess of the self than
technical skills? Furthermore, the outsider would hardly expect
the attention paid to moral performance given the prevailing
definitions of the professional as a technical expert who applies
a body of theoretic knowledge to perform certain functions valued
by the society in general (Parsons 1949, p. 372).

There is a third way in which controls of moral performance
are more conspicuous than controls of technical performance.
Controls of technical performance are "built into" the everyday
performance of tasks. Controls of moral performance are not.
They are quite extraordinary disturbances in group life at the
recurrent everyday level. They are characterized by the superordinate's assault on guilty parties. Public humiliations and dressing-downs, sarcastic and mock-ironic remarks, or a pointed

ignoring of the guilty party are all tactics superiors use to treat moral breaches. This all contrasts sharply with the handling of technical failure, for handling this failure blends into ongoing activity and seems a routine part of it. The manner in which a superordinate handles a moral lapse—his bracketing of the event as something memorable and distasteful—makes these breaches a more conspicuous feature of the environment than technical failures.

Perhaps the greater conspicuousness of moral error relative to technical error is merely an artifact of my research site, which is, after all, a training institution charged with the socialization of recruits. In the world of independent practice, this relationship would not hold up. This objection is an empirical one but empirically I do not have nor did I set out to gather the data to silence the objection. However, I do know that the number of technical errors is much greater than the number of disciplinary actions taken by hospital boards or state medical societies. I suspect that one reason for this is that for error to be considered culpable, technical failure must be wedded to a moral breach. Professionals restrict colleagues—and the extent of this restriction is for our particular purposes beside the point—for abusing the "good faith" requirement of professional action. The restriction of colleagues in other settings—its patterns and extent—is certainly a question for future research. Study of other medical settings and of other professions is of course needed. It would be foolhardy and wrong to argue that my site selection did not limit the generalizability of my data in any way. However, it also provided several advantages, the most important of which was to show professional controls in their most basic forms.

Forgiveness and Punishment

There is a second feature of group life that supports our contention that the control of techniques is subordinated to the control of morals: namely, there is a differential response to these breaches. Superordinates tend to be tolerant and forgiving of technical error and intolerant and unforgiving of moral error. This pattern of response shows us how moral competence acts as the organizing principle of a professional community.

Forgiveness and punishment of breaches are two mechanisms for establishing group membership or the boundaries of the professional group. The first is an inclusion mechanism; the second, one of exclusion. Distinct identity as a group depends on the operation of both mechanisms. If we are to understand the nature of a professional community, we need to look at both mechanisms.

Technical offenses are forgiven by superordinates. This leniency promotes cohesion among members of the work force. Forgiveness itself operates as a deterrence to further technical error. First, it obligates the subordinate who is forgiven to the superordinate who shows him mercy. To repay this obligation, the subordinate becomes more vigilant in the immediate future. Following a technical error, it is quite common for a subordinate to spend extra time with each patient on work rounds double-checking to make sure results are satisfactory. Second, when a subordinate sees his technical errors are forgiven, he recognizes that he has no incentive to hide them. He is less likely, therefore, to compound his problems by attempting to treat problems that are over his head for fear of superordinate reprisal. Forgiveness encourages "help-seeking" behavior and removes the stigma from uncertainty.

Forgiveness also serves to reintegrate offenders into the group. We see this most directly in the "hair-shirt" ritual that is part of the Mortality and Morbidity Conference. The self-criticism, confession, and forgiveness that are all part of this ceremony allow the offender to reenter the group. The "hair-shirt" ritual promotes group solidarity. In tightly knit communal groups such ceremonies are a regular part of group life. For example, forms of this practice are found in monasteries or the rural communes of China. "Hair-shirt" rituals are a form of public exorcism. Through them, whatever demons that led to incorrect practice are driven from the group.

There are parallels in the treatment of errors in technique by superordinates and subordinates. The houseofficer confesses to his attending. The attending confesses to the entire collegium, which is his superordinate. Both humble themselves and in turn both are forgiven and embraced. Forgiveness binds the confessor to the group and exacts a pledge from him to live up to standards in the future. Since in time all make errors in techniques, all are obliged in time to go before the group and humble themselves. Through this process of confession and forgiveness the group exacts the allegiance of all its members to its standards.

By the same token, the group can afford to be merciful in the face of technical error since its members openly confess them. First, such confession is ipso facto proof that an individual adheres to group standards and knows what the expectations for his behavior are. Second, such confessions serve as proof that an individual is punishing himself for his faults. Therefore, forgiveness serves to limit self-criticism and prevent an individual from being immobilized by guilt. Forgiveness helps individuals mobilize for action after failure has stripped them of a sense of mastery. Forgiveness helps individuals cope with the problematic features of medical practice. It is a necessary part of group life which sustains commitments and mobilizes actors in the face of inevitable failure.

Superordinate reaction to moral errors is severe and intolerant. Superordinates punish those who make moral errors. In the short run, they shame these individuals. The degradation of the subordinate who makes a moral error places him outside the group. The onus then falls on the subordinate to show that his lapse was only temporary and not representative of his work. He must show that he "has learned his lesson and been properly put in his place." Those who cannot demonstrate this in the long run are excommunicated from the group of surgeons at Pacific. Demonstrations that one has learned his place are signaled by increased deference to superordinate authority, greater attention to detail, and closer ties with nurses and patients. One makes a highly visible show to the superordinate that one is genuinely repentant.

Superordinate intervention and sanction are necessary for moral lapses but not for technical ones for a simple reason. When technical errors are made, the individual acknowledges his subordination to the group by the gesture of confession and self-criticism. He voluntarily humbles himself. He bows, lowers himself, in the face of group standards. This is not the case for moral errors. As we have seen, the cutting edge that defines moral errors is an individual's failure to acknowledge the underling status which the requirement of "good faith" behavior imposes. The failure to route problems properly because of professional pride or the failure to confess error and admit shortcomings— these are features of moral error but not of technical error. When he makes a moral error, the subordinate shows by his conduct that he does not acknowledge his subordination to the group and its standards. Under such conditions, the superordinate forcefully reminds him of this subordination. The anger that superordinates show on such occasions derives from the manner in which the subordinate has mocked the community and its values.

Just as the group can afford to be merciful in the face of technical error since an individual is contrite, submits himself to group authority, and pledges to do better, the group must be merciless in the face of moral error since an individual is prideful, contemptuous of the group's authority, and offers no assurance of future improvement. The authorities of the group must punish the offender in the second case since there is nothing that suggests the desire or resources for self-improvement. Moral errors disqualify one from civil treatment by the group. Such errors exclude one from the group. One is expected to learn quickly what is forbidden from the fierce response it evokes. Superordinates expect such behavior to be quickly extinguished. When the behavior is not extinguished in the individual, the individual is extinguished in the group.

Forgiveness and punishment are the poles of a continuum on which responses to deviant acts can be arrayed. Discussions of the function of deviance for group formation often emphasize one pole of the continuum to the exclusion of the other. For example, Bensman and Gerver (1963) discuss the importance that forgiving deviance in a factory has for creating group solidarity, while Erikson (1966) discusses the importance of punishment in Puritan New England for maintaining group identity. However, what both studies fail to appreciate fully is that both forgiveness and punishment are different sides of the same coin and that both are necessary if a group is to sustain a distinct identity and boundaries. The proper task of analysis is not to celebrate one process at the expense of the other, but rather to see which violations mobilize one mechanism and which mobilize the other. Forgiveness and punishment always coexist in different proportions in different communities at different times. The task of analysis is to explain these variations.

Corporate vs. Individual Self-Control

We are now in a position to state how professional self-control operates. Professionals forgive errors that are defined as involving techniques. The operations of control for these errors is inconspicuous; it is built into the everyday activities of the work group. Professionals punish errors that are defined as moral. The operation of controls is here quite conspicuous; it is set apart from everyday activities. This is to say that professionals interpret their mandate to control performance as an injunction to maintain a community of high moral standards. Those who show that they are unreliable, incapable of sacrifice, and unable to act in "good faith" in the patient's interest are excluded from the network of elite surgeons and granted only a limited mandate. Those who prove themselves reliable, capable of sacrifice, and able to act in "good faith" are invited into the elite professional network and granted an extensive mandate. In the control of work, technical performance is subordinated to moral performance. Simply stated, physicians do not expect the application of medical knowledge to be perfect. There will always be honest errors. However, physicians do expect perfect compliance with the norms of clinical responsibility. They see this compliance as their best defense and remedy for the honest and inevitable errors they will all occasionally make. Negligence is defined in terms of clinical norms—moral values—and not technical standards.

Unfortunately, we cannot allow matters to rest here. In the term *professional self control*, there is linguistic ambiguity. Read as *professional-self control*, it connotes the individual professional's ability to handle responsibility. It underscores the fact that the client can trust that the professional will restrain his own desire for gain and act in the client's interest. When the emphasis is on the professional-self, the term celebrates the moral stature to which the individual has grown. Read as *professional self-control*, the term underscores the corporate responsibility of the profession to regulate its own internal affairs. This reading emphasizes the contract between the profession and lay society. The ambiguity of the term reflects an underlying ambiguity over the interpretation of license and mandate. We cannot make clear with a hyphen what is an inherently problematic feature of social life.

However, we can point out problems raised by this ambiguity by juxtaposing these two different readings of *professional self control*. From the emphasis in the education of surgeons on character building and the moral development of surgeons, it is clear that the profession places much weight on prefessional self-control, or the individual's control of his professional self. As superordinates see it, the goal of training is to turn out, after five years, individuals with the capacity to display this professional-self control. We know that education is an imperfect mechanism of social control and that not everyone develops this control. We have seen that those who do not develop these controls are downwardly mobile in professional networks. The question becomes: Who or what controls these individuals as they pursue their careers? What does the corporate control of individual professionals look like when viewed in a setting less exclusive than Pacific Hospital and across settings for the profession as a whole? We do know of the hesitancy of the profession to establish standards which discriminate unacceptable from acceptable performance and of the well-documented tendency (Friedson and Rhea 1972; cf. also chapter 5 above) of the profession to punish by exclusion, thus protecting a few professionals but hardly lay society from less than adequate performance. This suggests to us that there is a hypertrophy of professional-self control and an atrophy of professional self-control.

The hypertrophy of individual self-control and the atrophy of corporate self-control becomes all the more apparent when we focus on the surgery department rather than on the individual service as the unit of analysis, when we look more closely at quasi-normative errors, and when we examine the reactions of the surgeons at Pacific to the "dumps" of their colleagues at other institutions. Analyzing controls on a service, we find a system in which attendings exercise authority without hesitation. Subordinates' errors are discovered and corrected by superordinates. If the error is technical or judgmental, sanctions are restitutive; actions are taken to restore the situation to normal. If the error is normative or quasi-normative, sanctions are repressive; actions are taken which punish the guilty party. In this ritual drama of social control, housestaff and attendings never exchange roles. Superordinates discover breaches and they discover them of subordinates and never of each other. These interactive patterns do not mean that attending surgeons are such moral and technical virtuosos that they never commit breaches which offend the sensibilities of colleagues or even of subordinates. Rather, these patterns speak to the symbolic importance of the completion of training and to the attainment of staff position as a form of moral licensing. Further, such patterns indicate how firmly the norm of autonomy is embedded in medical culture. On a surgical service, professional controls exist in a hierarchical relationship composed of one set of subordinates and two superordinates who are some-what independent of each other. The domain of social control is limited; each service is a self-consciously isolated unit. The boundaries of the authority system are the scope of each attending's authority. For all intents and purposes these boundaries are never breached. Attending surgeons do not meddle in each other's affairs, unless explicitly asked for advice on a case, or unless making a dramatic gesture of deference to another attending such as first-assisting in a procedure to learn a new technique. At all other times, the respect and freedom which attendings accord each other in organizing their services gives controls their self-consciously isolated quality. Services, then, are the locus of control and not the department. What from one perspective is a detailed and harsh system of controls is, from another, a system in which corporate responsibility is virtually absent and in which individuals are given great license. Within the surgery department at Pacific, quality of care is almost totally dependent on the skills and conscience of individual practitioners and almost independent of any structural constraints save that of hierarchy. Here it is important to remember that a formal hierarchy does not observably govern interaction among attendings on different services the way that it constrains the behavior of individuals on specific services. Individuals on services act within a well-defined hierarchy, while individuals at a departmental level do not. However well behavior is controlled at the service level, at the department level there are no formal devices, save the Mortality and Morbidity Conference, to ensure a uniform quality of care. The Mortality and Morbidity Conference is, of course, a retrospective review of behavior. The surgery department at Pacific, with its highly elaborated conception of autonomy, individual self-control, and its relative absence of corporate controls, is an exquisite miniature of the way medical controls work in general (Freidson 1975).

Rather than merely decry this state of affairs, we are in a position to explain why individual conscience is so well articulated as a control and why corporate devices are so underdeveloped. An understanding of two key mechanisms is crucial here: (1) the attending's authority and (2) quasi-normative error. We have described each service as an independent authority system with the boundaries consisting of the attending's authority. The attending's authority rests on his legal responsibility to the patient. The physician's fiduciary trust is not just a feature of sociological description, it is also embedded within our legal system. So, despite the fact that he makes many of the everyday treatment decisions and that he is responsible for much of the service's operation, the subordinate in a legal sense has no autonomy. He is merely an extension of the attending. When an attending punishes a houseofficer, he is punishing his subordinate as an appendage of himself, as his representative to the patient. In disciplining a houseofficer, the attending is displaying the invisible standards he applies to himself. The superordinate-subordinate relationship permits the dramaturgical depiction of conscience at very little cost to the superordinate. The authority of the attending rests here on his right to care for patients in the manner that he deems proper. This is a power that the house-officer cannot yet claim because he has not yet earned it. He does not have a full professional self. License, the granting of the great personal autonomy, the giving of the right of individuality to the professional himself, is awarded only after training is completed. An attending feels free to reprimand houseofficers as if they were children and often for no better reason than "I'm the boss and that's the way I want things done," for the houseofficer has not passed fully through the sets of rites, rituals, and ordeals that transform outsiders into insiders and make colleagues out of subordinates. But the crucial point is: once such a transformation occurs, a professional self is seen as something inviolable. Corporate responsibility is discharged through the socialization and education of recruits. Just as it is inappropriate for parents to meddle in the lives of their grown children, surgeons view meddling as inappropriate surveillance of the performance of those released from training. In a way, the attending position on social control may be characterized as follows: For the five years they are home—while they are housestaff—you work hard with them, you try to provide a good environment, you send them out and you hope for the best. The corporate responsibility of the profession is not seen to extend beyond raising one generation of surgeons after another from professional infancy to professional adulthood.

However, as in any socialization period that takes a substantial portion of time, the relations among the generations is marked by conflict. Quasi-normative errors as a symbolization of this inequality among the generations allow us to understand this conflict more fully. A complete professional self is one that has earned the right to organize its work in a manner that it sees fit. This right belongs to attendings; it does not yet belong to houseofficers, although they often claim it. Quasi-normative errors act on two distinct levels as boundary-maintaining devices that uphold the privileges of rank for attendings. First, such idiosyncratic standards of proper practice establish the right of the attendings on each service to employ their own best judgment in carrying out their work. What it is "wrong" for housestaff to do on one service, an attending on another service may do as a matter of standard procedure. The judgment, maturity, honesty, and suitability for a surgical career of a houseofficer who makes repeated quasi-normative errors would be open to question. Yet attending A and attending B view the differences between themselves as nothing more than an artifact of training, clinical experience, individual philosophy, personality—in a word, as a difference in style. In this setting, differences of style among colleagues are recognized as legitimate. To reduce many matters of disagreement about proper practice to questions of style removes them as a serious topic for discussion, or possibly control. For while one may like or dislike a style, one very rarely finds in a style cause for moral outrage and social control. That large area surgeons relegate to style when evaluating one another (and error when judging subordinates) serves to underscore their autonomy as professionals while diminishing the range of practices seen as open to public debate and control. Quasi-normative errors—that is, the stylistic idiosyncracies of attendings—serve to isolate the surgical services from one another.

Second, and perhaps in the long run more significant, is the way quasi-normative error serves as a device to maintain the boundary between attending and housestaff. The attending has the power to impose his will on a situation whatever the merits of the arguments a houseofficer may muster to defend his course of action. At an everyday level, events treated as matters of style among colleagues are treated as matters of morals between ranks. The fact that attendings react in a similar fashion to normative errors, where there is consensus within the collegium, and also react similarly to quasi-normative errors where there is no consensus, may have several regrettable consequences. It may mean, in the first place, that the moral lessons of normative error have not been properly internalized. Housestaff mistakenly link similarities of response to similarities of stimulus and confuse genuine norms with quasi-norms. They treat all repressive sanction as flowing from the arbitrary, capricious, dogmatic, and unreasonably autocratic personalities of attendings rather than from deeply held common sentiments shared by a community of fellow surgeons. In this case, they would be unable to develop strong commitments to the community norms since they would be unable to perceive that such norms exist. All shortcomings become attributable to personality and style. In the second place, the treatment of quasi-normative error cultivates in housestaff an appreciation for the pains of subordination. The completion of training signifies being out from under. The houseofficer, in talking about the future of a prospective surgeon, emphasizes his freedom to make his own decisions, his freedom from others' eccentricities, and his freedom from the opinions of others. Here, quasi-normative error weakens a future surgeon's ties to a colleague community and at the same time fails to instill a finely etched sense of what constitutes good and bad practice. Independence, freedom, and professional autonomy become completely egoistic; the ritual passage of residency can fail to transmit the culture to the recruit. Furthermore, quasi-normative error serves as a gloss for attendings to lean on the authority of their office rather than their expertise. Labeling a behavior a quasi-normative error closes off discussion of its appropriateness without an assessment of its merits. Such labeling prevents the give-and-take necessary to keep attendings sharp. Finally, quasi-normative error can depress housestaff initiative and zeal and thereby encourage the mindless following of routines.

The behavior of the surgeons at Pacific to the "dumps" of colleagues elsewhere is yet another indicator of how undeveloped corporate responsibility is within the profession. "Dumps" are mismanaged patients sent to Pacific from other hospitals. Basically, surgeons do not publicly condemn or reprimand the most outrageous performances. Their rationale is twofold: (1) if the surgeon is a responsible, ethical colleague, he knows he has made a hash out of the case, so there is, as the surgeons say, "no reason to rub his nose in it"; or, alternatively, if he is not responsible and ethically competent, then the dumping surgeon is a "bandit" and nothing anyone says will change him; and (2) either way one has it, if one complains and makes "dumping" unpleasant and difficult for the surgeon in trouble, he would rather bury his problems before suffering the "bad manners" of Pacific staff and seeking help for them. Silence, then, is seen as the response that best protects patients. At Pacific, the response of superordinates to "dumps" is to crack the whip harder over the heads of their subordinates in the hope that negligence is a generational problem and that their redoubled efforts to establish professional-self controls, a well-articulated sense of individual responsibility, will eradicate such lackadaisical behaviors. All the while, the attendings at Pacific fail to instill such controls in some subordinates and release them from training—and from their watchful eyes—to send dumps to Pacific in the future. The problem is not, as some have claimed (Barber et al. 1973; Gray 1975; Crane 1975) an absence of any socialization, controls, or ethical sense in the profession; the problem is rather a system which celebrates individual conscience as a control while ignoring corporate responsibility. The profession of medicine needs to develop structural remedies—or structure socialization—in a way that brings into balance both the corporate and the individual dimensions of control. Adequate controls in the profession exist only to the degree that a corporate moral sense is cultivated equal to the individual moral sense.

Summing Up

In this report we have described the system of controls that regulates behavior among surgeons. We have discovered what these controls are, how they are enforced, how they have far-reaching consequences for channeling fledgling surgeons into different career paths, and how these standards are learned by subordinates. We have seen why the controls which do obtain in the profession are so uneven. Being matters of conscience, they may be very strongly internalized by individuals or they may be only weakly present.

The findings of this report differ from those of others in ways that should be made clear. First, Freidson (1970) and others who follow him emphasize the hesitation with which controls operate and the mildness of most punishments. The position of those who emphasize "professional dominance" give sociological credence to Shaw's famous dictum that "all professions are conspiracies against the laity." We have found, however, that these patterns cannot be explained adequately as maneuvers by the profession to retain a stranglehold on the market. What we have found is that the hesitation and mildness which surrounds controls are best understood in light of the way a surgeon's knowledge about the world is structured. The uncertainty which the surgeon routinely faces in making a diagnosis and pinpointing a precise causative agent for therapeutic misadventure accounts for a great deal when explaining why surgeons discipline errant colleagues as they do and when explaining why normative rather than technical breaches are the more serious errors. In short, in understanding social control in a profession I feel it is best not to stray too far from the cognitive frameworks the profession itself employs to make sense of the world. To take the role of the other impels us to look at how the other constructs his world. We need to know which objects in this world are taken for granted, which are problematic, and which are considered irrelevant for the purposes at hand. If, in the study of lower-class deviance, it is unwarrantable to bootleg everyday definitions of right and wrong into our work, it is just as inadmissable to do so in the case of high-status professionals. One of the strengths of this report, not common in other works in the field, is that it attempts to take the sociology of knowledge of modern medicine seriously, the better to see how the nature of a particular cognitive realm structures values, attitudes, and practice with regard to error. A sophisticated sociology of medicine must have some familiarity with, at the very least, the nature of medical reasoning in order to appreciate the coded language in which colleagues raise questions, communicate approval, shoulder blame, and hurl accusations at each other. I am not saying that all studies in the sociology of medicine should necessarily display this understanding of the physician's phenomenal world; I am saying only that we need to place a greater emphasis on such understanding in the future than we have in the past. As sociologists, it is peculiar that we have such appreciation for the "symbolic" interaction and linguistic codes of corner boys, prostitutes, drug users, fences, members of communes, and so on, and so little appreciation of and tolerance for the same dimensions of action among physicians.

The recent work of Barber, Crane, and Gray claims that physicians receive almost no ethical training through their socialization. My claim is that postgraduate training of surgeons is above all things an ethical training. Subordinates are harshly disciplined when they violate the ethical standards of the discipline. They are promoted and accepted into the ranks as colleagues on the basis of their ethical fitness. It is true that the moral standards demanded and the superordinate's self-interest converge here to a great degree. Nevertheless, the point remains that normative standards of dedication, interest, and thoroughness are applied in evaluating subordinates rather than narrowly technical standards. Moreover, ethical dilemmas such as how to most appropriately manage the terminal patient are discussed during rounds. The moral and ethical dimensions of training are not bracketed from all other concerns but are instead built into everyday clinical life. It is unwarrantable to infer from absence of formal courses, seminars, and so on that ethical "training" is relegated merely to the informal structure of role learning. Perhaps one of the reasons that Barber, Crane, and Gray missed the ethical dimension of training is that their survey research methodology is too distant from the rhythms of everyday life to capture this dimension of action. Time and again surgeons express their feelings by indirection—the horror story is a good example. To understand how surgeons debate ethical concerns requires knowledge of that same coded language surgeons use to discuss error. I am not suggesting that sociological analysis is a subtle, new form of mysticism which requires a divining of the real meaning lurking beneath the surface of interaction. On the contrary, I suggest that sociological analysis begins with an understanding of what actors mean when they talk to each other. Such knowledge requires a respect for the word and gesture as units of social meaning, a respect that rests on our understanding of the *gestalt* which structures any word's meaning. Since we expect each occupation to have a unique *gestalt* based on its typical work problems, we expect members of occupational groups to speak to each other in their own coded ways. To learn the language of an occupational group, to learn its ways, we need to spend time observing how they meet the routine contingencies of the workplace.

Once we learn the ways workers speak to each other in the workplace, we see things that were previously obscure. A third difference in this report from others concerns the nature of in-group solidarity among professionals. We commonly believe that physicians maintain a conspiracy of silence, protecting incompetent colleagues by shielding their mistakes from the lay public. This account makes clear that this silence is not merely a feature of professional-client relations, but that it is also a feature of the public confessional, the Mortality and Morbidity Conference. When an attending "puts on the hair shirt," he takes blanket responsibility for a case. He maintains a conspiracy of silence. He does not publicly announce which subordinates made which errors. The in-group solidarity of the service as a working group would be crushed by such an open betrayal of its confidences. In a sense, Mortality and Morbidity Conferences such as Pacific's serve as a model of the lesson "we don't tell tales" as well as "we openly admit our mistakes and strive to correct them." Conspiracies of silence are not in and of themselves evil things. They are, however, harmful when they allow a group to practice without any incentives to curb their excesses. A problem exists for the profession of medicine when the lessons of silence are learned without the concomitant lesson that the professional himself has the responsibility to correct his errors. Professional responsibility is itself thought of as individual and not corporate responsibility.

This last point leads me to make a concluding recommendation. I feel that improved performance is desirable, necessary and possible in the social control of medicine. Such performance rests on the profession's developing a corporate sense equal to its individual sense. While it is impossible to specify, in a step-by-step fashion, a program for accomplishing this, my account makes clear what elements contribute to an effective control system. First, there must be some hierarchy, or a functional equivalent, that permits question-answer sequences, what we call the competence quizzes of rounds, about the appropriateness of different treatment modalities. Second, some face-to-face interaction is necessary. Physicians need to feel part of the same community and answerable to one another. Third, there must be public forums for discussing problems and allocating blame. Such forums create as well as sustain a community by giving members a sense of their shared identity. Fourth, the community needs some control of sanctions so that it is able to control malefactors within its own ranks. The dilemmas involved in handling "dumps," or in dismissing subordinates from Pacific only to lose the capacity to restrain them, need resolution. At present, a physician's conscience is not only his guide but the patient's only protection. The patient deserves the protection of not only the individual's but also the collectivity's conscience. Beyond that, the profession as a whole needs to raise its conscience about its public responsibilities. The collectivity needs to promote the structural changes that will build stronger accounting mechanisms into everyday practice.

Appendix

The Field-Worker and
the Surgeon

All fieldwork done by a single field-worker invites the question, Why should we believe it? It would be nice to be able to claim that I was a totally impartial observer whose characteristic ways of looking at the world allow an almost perfect mirroring of some objective reality. However, as the fieldwork experience made clear to me, I am not without my biases. I would like to pretend that this was not so for any number of reasons, but the observer role in some sense trained me to see these biases in a heightened way. As I reflect on the experience of eighteen months of participant observation in a teaching hospital, and on the dilemmas of the observer role, I feel a sense of respect for data-collecting procedures which allow the researcher to keep the sensuous world at a distance, and which thereby allow him to avoid the self-exposure, self-reflection, and self-doubt endemic to field-workers. In the field, the everyday life of his subjects overwhelms the researcher, threatens to obliterate his sense of self, and forces a reconsideration of deeply held personal and intellectual beliefs. It would be of little point, then, for me to pretend in the face of such a powerful experience that I was merely a coding machine which transcribed the events of everyday life first into field material and then into the sociological and literary order of the preceding pages. In this appendix, I would like to describe the field experience itself and the analysis of the data. This appendix should show the reader how I identified and controlled for my own biases and should allow him to control for them independently of me.

In the Field

How did I begin? The first thing I did was to approach an attending I had met at a party, explain my proposed study, and ask for his cooperation. The attending expressed enthusiasm for the project, but refused his cooperation. He claimed that if I wanted to really be trusted, I would need the housestaff's acceptance. He expressed his fear that his sponsorship would be a "kiss of death": housestaff would view me as his spy and never talk freely with me. If I wanted my project to succeed, he advised, I needed to be seen as my own person. So rather than somehow magically start the research, he gave me the names of a number of residents and the hospital's central page number. What I learned during this interview was that there was no instant access for the field-worker. Not sure if I was receiving aid or a runaround from my initial contact, I called the first name on his list, the chief resident. We met for coffee and I explained my plans. The resident approved my being an observer on his service, but claimed he would have to check with both attendings. The chairman of my department provided a letter of introduction to the chairman of the Department of Surgery. Gaining my initial entrée was a multistaged diplomatic problem. Each interaction was a test, and access was the result of continual testing and retesting. Entrée was not something negotiated once and then over and done with. I was always entering new scenes and situations involving different combinations of people. Fortunately, of course, I could rely on what I had learned in previous encounters and the repertoire of roles that I had developed and that others developed for me. The important thing that field-workers must keep in mind is that entrée is not a single event but a continuous process.

Access—being allowed in the scene—is one thing, but approval and trust of field subjects is quite another. Just like access, cooperation cannot be ordered by fiat, but is rather earned again and again, when the field-worker shows that he or she is trustworthy and reliable. Much is made in fieldwork accounts of the "cover story" which the observer uses to explain his presence in the setting as a first and essential step in gaining trust. My cover story was very simple. I explained that I was doing a dissertation on the way surgeons learned to recognize and control error. The surgeons were, as a rule, remarkably uncurious about my research. None ever questioned the legitimacy of my research question or the nature of my methods during our initial meetings. Few even requested that I account for my presence. I was not asked for my cover story very often and, when asked for the story, I was not required to elaborate on it. In some sense, my access was secured by sponsorship of housestaff trusted by all. Once my access was established, my cover story was superfluous and served as a gloss during introductions. In the everyday course of things, my housestaff sponsor was more important to my access than any cover story I used.

Trust was gained neither during initial introductions nor by the artful manipulation of a cover story, but through my performance in roles I assumed and was assigned by housestaff and attendings. Housestaff assigned me a number of roles. Most generally, I was an "extra pair of hands," and a "gofer." During the time of my fieldwork, I became very proficient at opening packages of bandages, retrieving charts, and fetching items from the supply room. Through these tasks, I expressed some solidarity with whatever group I was observing and gave something, however inconsequential, in exchange for "observing rights." Second, I was an "emissary from the outside world." My round of life was less circumscribed than a houseofficer's: I read and watched more news, saw more movies, and participated more fully in university life outside the hospital. In some sense, I provided housestaff contact with a world they felt cut off from. During Watergate, I always brought a number of papers into the hospital. How or why this became my task I do not know. Often I purchased these papers at the hospital gift stand, a place interns and residents certainly had access to. Their general reluctance to pick such papers up is not so much a mark of their frugality as a symbolic statement about their relation to the world outside Pacific Hospital. I later learned that housestaff attach a magical property to newspapers, books, and magazines. If they bring them in to work they see this as jinxing themselves and condemning the group to an impossible busy day. It is, however, permissible for outsiders to bring such taboo items to them. My passing remarks about movies, current events, the weather—all were taken as an indication of what educated people on the outside were thinking. Third, I was a "fellow-sufferer." As a graduate student not released from training, I was perceived as occupying a position analagous to the houseofficer's. My own career problems and expectations were topics that houseofficers initiated much conversation about. They constantly compared and contrasted our different experiences. During such exchanges, houseofficers constantly emphasized the indignity of their roles and often suggested that their present burdens justified their future rewards. From me, they sought to learn about the generalized indignities of the subordinate role in sociological training. I regaled them with my wildest recollections of coding data and proofreading galleys.

Fourth, I was a convenient "sounding board." I was surprised at the degree that informants sought me out to relate stories of practice that they disagreed with. Feelings that were not shared in the group, discontents, uncertainties were taken to me. I knew that observers were often sought by organizational malcontents; what surprised me was that all my informants were at one time or another malcontents. Such a label was not a stable organizational identity as much as a fleeting reaction to behavior, which for one reason or another offended the houseofficer's sensibilities. Disfiguring palliative operations, patient discomfort, and the openness of communications among the ranks were the most common complaints. As a "sounding board," I was implicitly asked to play a quasi-therapeutic role: to listen without judging and to understand. The fact that I was asked to play this role so often by so many speaks both to their understanding of what an observer does and to the deep feelings that physicians repress as a matter of course. As a rule, we, as medical sociologists, have not concentrated enough on how fragile physician defenses are, what events disturb them, and how primal the existential material they are dealing with is. Birth, life, death are not questions that one works through definitively. We need to pay more attention to the provisional nature of the resolution physicians make to the conflicts such subjects present. My own graduate students in the field now report that their informants ask them to play this quasi-

therapeutic role, also. Like me, they find it both disturbing and
flattering. The fact that our subjects choose to use us in this way
suggests both that we need to learn methods for containing and
managing these encounters, and also that we cannot define the
field-worker role totally in instrumental terms. We come to have
identities for our subjects quite independent of the ones we
promote for ourselves. Ironically, it is often these identities that
yield the greatest amount of data.

Fifth, houseofficers viewed me as a "referee" in conflicts
among themselves over patient management, quarrels over the
equity of the division of labor, and disputes about whether or not
patients understood what was happening. In the midst of such
disagreements, one houseofficer would turn to me and ask:
"Well, what do you think? Which of us is right?" These were not
comfortable situations for me when I could hide behind the
observer role. A judgment was demanded as the price for my
continued presence. Moreover, any judgment was certain to
alienate one of my informants. I developed tactics for throwing
the question back to the disputants or for pointing out the merits
of either side, or making a joke of the entire dispute. Over time, I
tried in vain to teach my subjects that such conflict resolution was
not a proper part of my role. Nevertheless, being asked to referee
disputes was a recurrent and always problematic task and not one
that I ever felt totally comfortable with. As I felt more accepted, I
was somewhat better able to put questions off. But in the beginning, I was stiff, uncomfortable, and always mindful of my relationships with each party. As a referee, I was able to elicit good
material when I was able to turn the dispute into an occasion for
discussing different attitudes and beliefs toward medical practice.
Unfortunately, I was not always levelheaded enough to accomplish this because I felt so put-on-the-spot by such confrontations.

Sixth, I was the group "historian." Because of the way housestaff rotate through the various services, it was not unusual for me
to have been on either the Able or the Baker Service longer than
any particular houseofficer. When this occurred, I was expected
to know something of the history of the different patients on the
service. I was expected to keep track of attendings' remarks and

verify them for absent group members. The role of group historian served me well, since it forced housestaff to depend on me for information that they needed. This created a greater sense of mutual obligation between housestaff and myself and to the degree that the information I supplied was reliable, I established my credibility. Also, I was a short-run as well as long-run historian. I would often ask housestaff about action that I could not watch but was interested in. (Much work is done individually, and on any given day I saw only a portion of possible action.) On more than one occasion, my questioning reminded houseofficers of a task that had until then slipped their minds. My unwitting reminders saved them from oversights which would have gotten them into trouble. The fact that such incidents occurred further indebted housestaff to me and heightened my legitimacy. A field-worker pays a price for this kind of legitimacy, though. The historian role itself presents some of the most common moral dilemmas that a field-worker faces. Each time I gave such a reminder to a houseofficer, I changed what would have otherwise happened without this intervention. Lab tests, consultations with other physicians, and conferences with patients and their families—all these were on occasion events that took place because I reminded houseofficers of them. By jogging the memory of house-officers in this way, I made it impossible for myself to observe what happens when these events fail to occur. On these occasions, I did not intend to alter the natural course of events; but it did happen that I unwittingly created an occasional participant-observer effect.

Despite the fact that it was not my intention in these instances to change the action I was studying, one can see very clearly that errors of omission present the observer with a moral dilemma. If one does remind a houseofficer, one disturbs by that act the very relationships one is attempting to study. However, if one does not remind the houseofficer—and yet knows he has overlooked something—it is possible that a patient's care will be compromised. On most cases when I asked if something had been done, I did so because as a sociologist I was particularly interested in seeing or hearing a report of that specific action, and usually because I was

unaware of whether it had occurred or not—I was trying to orient
myself. If the houseofficer had forgotten about the task I was
asking about, if it had completely slipped his mind, then that fact
told me something about the difference between a sociological
perspective and a surgical one; and I learned something more
about the structure of the surgeon's life-world. There was one
category of event, however—conferences with patients and
families—that I asked about more than others. Here I was often
conscious of my participation in the scene, but thought that some
patients (exactly which patients these were and why I reacted to
them the way I did is a complex matter that I do not understand)
deserved fuller explanations than they often got from the surgeons. A question that I cannot answer is, Did the surgeons see
my role as a sociologist such that they presumed that I was
interested in such group phenomena, and did they come to rely on
me to remind them of their diffuse obligations to patients and
their families? Is this the major role they assigned me in the
group? If it was, who was responsible for making sure that this
team responsibility was filled when there was no sociologist
present? Whatever the answers to these questions, a rule of
thumb I applied was to keep my reminders as few as possible.
This was a rule I occasionally broke because of my feelings for a
patient and his/her family. I must also confess to one other
category of event on which I routinely broke my own rule. As a
group historian, I occasionally asked questions that served as
reminders to subjects that I felt were hostile and/or skeptical of
my sociological enterprise to establish that I belonged in the field;
that I was concerned, aware and helpful; and that I was a
legitimate member of the group. The fact is I occasionally used
my questions to demonstrate the ways the group needed me. (One
could also argue at the same time I was proving to myself that I
served some useful purpose in the group.)

   If errors of omission present observers with one type of moral
dilemma, errors of commission present him with another. In the
case where the field-worker knows that some harm has been done
to a patient through physician or nursing error, does the observer
have any direct, ethical obligations to the patient and his/her

family? That is, should the field-worker either inform the patient or find some alternative means of making public the error? I chose not to do this for a variety of reasons. As a pragmatic matter, being a patient-advocate would have made the kind of fieldwork I wanted to do impossible. Moreover, I felt a responsibility to other medical sociologists who wished to undertake field projects in the future. I was aware that my conduct could either make the way more or less difficult for those who followed me. While some participant-observer effects seem acceptable to me, others, those that contravene the basic operating norms of a group, are not acceptable. These larger effects not only distort the phenomenon under study, they make it impossible for later field-workers to gain access to and legitimacy within medical settings. Most important, I felt I could discharge my ethical obligations to patients more effectively by describing the general categorization and management of error rather than tilting at windmills in one or two select cases. On the face of it, this kind of advocacy would not seem to be much of a problem; in fact, it is hard to imagine a field-worker, insistent on imposing his definitions of justice on a scene, completing his work. However, this fact is not as significant as the importance of recognizing the strong feelings that observing in a hospital evokes, and restraining the "rescuer" impulses that witnessing so much pain, suffering, and death provokes. Whatever roles houseofficers cast me in or I assumed, the major irony of the field-worker role was always apparent: on the one hand, I was intimately involved in all aspects of the everyday life of a group; and on the other hand, I was constrained by the nature of my task to exert as little social influence in that group as possible. So, my sensitivity to the group's actions and their consequences was heightened at the same time that my theoretic commitments restrained me from even raising the group's consciousness about the effects of its own actions.

I had less intimate contact with attendings than with house-staff, and assumed and was assigned a narrower range of roles. Most commonly, I was seen as any other "medical student." Attendings assimilated me to the group by treating me like any other member of the group. They had me look down proctoscopy tubes, rake abdomens feeling for a mass, and learn to hold retractors properly. Their treatment of me helped strengthen my ties to houseofficers, who saw that not only was I not in league with attendings, but that, like them, I was the occasional butt of an attending's sense of humor. By the same token, my own willingness to take part this way in group life served notice to attendings that I was willing to do what was necessary to complete my project. When attendings viewed me as a medical student, they often tried to teach me concise medical lessons. Whatever problems of identification and rapport I might have had, it is interesting to note that attendings had some of their own. Toward the end of my fieldwork, two attendings approached me, told me that I must be interested in medicine to have spent so much time at Pacific, and then informed me that if I wanted to go to medical school, they would help me in any way they could. I took their offer as an indication that perhaps I had been in the field long enough.

The incident above is related to another role attendings cast me in—their "advisee." Attendings offered two types of advice. First, there was "scientific" advice. Here attendings would address themselves to the design of my study. They wanted to know about my control groups, my measurement instruments, my hypotheses, and all similar paraphernalia from the type of research they engaged in. When I would explain that my model for research was somewhat different than theirs, they were skeptical but generally tolerant. After all, I was the sociology department's problem, and not theirs. Second, attendings offered "interpretive advice." When we were alone, they would often explain why they acted in certain situations the way they did, what they felt to be the burdens of their authority, what the major problems doing surgery in a major medical center were, what the personal strengths and weaknesses of their colleagues were, and so on. Like houseofficers (although the opportunity arose less frequently), attendings unloaded themselves on me. It is worth noting here that I was ten years younger than the youngest attending, so the fact that they used me as a "sounding board" points to ways in which the surgeon's role remains disturbing even to those who have practiced it all of their adult lives.

In addition, attendings used me often as a "clown" to diffuse tensions in the group. When things were going poorly, attendings on occasion would question me like any other member of the group and then poke fun at my fumbling and ignorance. Sitting around the doctors' lounge, the rigors of academic life would be compared unfavorably with those of surgery; and my manly virtues would be impugned. It was not always as a clown that attendings used me to ease tensions. Just as with housestaff, I was asked to referee conflict. My study was used by them to deflect conversations from their course. So that often when faced with troublesome questions from nurses or other physicians, they would give a noncommittal response and then ask me to explain my study. They would ply me with questions until they were sure the conversation could safely resume. These three roles were not assumed with equal frequency nor were all assumed from the first day of fieldwork. From the beginning and most generally, I was assimilated as a medical student. Then I was used as a "diffuser of tensions." If I passed the test implied in this role, I became an occasional confidant of the attending. With one attending who was not greatly invested in clinical issues, I was never other than a quasi-medical student. With the others, I played all three roles, albeit with varying frequency and intensity.

So far in this description I have concentrated on the various roles I played in the field setting. The rationale for this is simple. In the analysis of our fieldwork data, we concentrate on the role relations among participants in the scene we choose to study. Yet we often pay comparatively less attention to our own role relations with the subjects who make our knowledge of the setting and of the action possible. Since in fieldwork these relationships are our major methodological tool, they require serious discussion. How we manage these relationships determines the depth, validity, and reliability of the data we collect and the inferences we draw from it. We need devices that ensure control of our like and dislike of various participants, the weighting that we give

incidents, and the ways our own everyday roles impinge on and
create strains with the field-worker role. The problem of objective
description and analysis is in itself formidable even if one were
only observing a television program, for example. In fieldwork,
the problem is made more complex because of the deep relationships and attachments one builds over time to one's subjects. As
Charles Lidz (1977) has correctly pointed out, the right and
privilege of being an observer is a gift presented to the researcher
by his host and subjects. So the observer has, in addition to
whatever the other problems that becloud his structured role-
relations with his subjects, the very special problems that attend
the giving and receiving of gifts. I would agree with Lidz that the
recognition and proper understanding of the gift relationship
serves as both a convenient theoretical framework for understanding the peculiar dilemmas of the field-worker and at the
same time a formidable restraint on bias in observation and
interpretation.

First, what are the special features of the gift relationship? As
Mauss (1967) pointed out in his classic statement, the giver and
the recipient of a gift are involved in an interactional sequence
that involves giving, receiving, and reciprocating. Even more
important, involvement in a gift cycle creates a solidarity among
participants and signifies that they have obligations toward each
other that extend into the future. The fact that the field-worker is
both the receiver of a gift and a guest means that he has a diffuse
sense of obligation to his host-giver-subject. Field-workers have
long recognized their indebtedness to their subjects. In fact, as
one reads accounts of fieldwork itself one senses that this burden
is truly "the magnificient obsession" of those who employ this
research method. While not explicitly analyzing the observer role
as a gift relationship, field-workers worry, in their writings, over
fulfilling their obligations to their subjects, over balancing personal debts to individuals against universal debts to the discipline
of sociology, and over discharging obligations to subjects that
extend beyond the life of any particular piece of research. In
addition, there is the field-worker's typical ethical dilemma: what
if the data I gather are potentially harmful to my subjects? What

if the facts themselves betray those to whom I have become so attached over so many months? Others have spoken of the "tyranny of the gift" in different contexts, but it is clear that the gift of access, of witnessing social life as it is lived in someone else's environment, exercises a tyranny of its own. This tyranny has as its most distinctive features three significant elements: (1) the danger of overrapport, so thoroughly merging with the subject's point of view that one cannot achieve the critical distance necessary for analysis; (2) the danger of overindebtedness, so thoroughly feeling a sense of diffuse obligation that one can no longer assess what one does and does not properly owe his subjects; and (3) the danger of overgeneralization, so thoroughly idealizing one's subjects that one sees their behavior as overly representative of all persons in a class.

I was protected from overrapport and overindebtedness in part by the very structure of hospital life. Unlike field-workers who spend years with an unchanging population, my subjects rotated through the surgical services fairly rapidly. Some stayed for as little as a month; none stayed over three months. There were housestaff I liked very much; housestaff I detested; and others I barely got to know. Whatever the case, there was an unending parade of housestaff. The mere fact that I was observing so many people in rapid succession prevented overrapport with any one subject. There was, of course, the danger that I would identify with the structural position of being a houseofficer, even if I avoided strong attachments to specific individuals. After all, I was a twenty-four-year-old graduate student, subordinate to a dissertation committee, and struggling to achieve autonomy within my own profession. Surely there was a clear and ever-present danger that, being a subordinate myself, I would overidentify with the subordinate and his problems. Overrapport with housestaff was avoided by two features of my everyday life. First, my wife, Marjorie Waxman, was supervising child-care workers in a psychiatric hospital at the time of this research. My conversations with her made me sensitive to the problems of the superordinate, especially the difficulty of balancing the needs of patient care with the needs of subordinates to develop their own skills and judgments through their own mistakes. Second, my major field-supervisor constantly pointed out to me instances when I seemed to take subordinate complaints too much to heart and urged me to see beyond the specific perturbations in housestaff-attending relations to see what are generic problems in superordinate-subordinate relations. Of course, I also had to guard against the opposite problem, overidentification with attendings. After all, did they not have, to an exaggerated degree, the autonomy I was working so hard to obtain? Here, I was protected from over-rapport by a number of factors. First, my relations with attendings were not as regular, intense, or relaxed as those with housestaff. Second, several of my own friends in medical training served as constant reminders of the subordinate's problem. Third, there is a general resistance in sociology to sympathize with the perspec-tive of authority. Authors such as Becker (1970) constantly remind us whose side we should be on.

My resolution to the problem of overindebtedness was some-what different than the resolution to overrapport, and unfolded over time in two quite separate phases. A moderately sensitive observer of life in the surgery wards of a hospital will be flooded with feelings of helplessness. These feelings themselves have two distinct components. First, witnessing so much pain and suf-fering, the field-worker wants to roll up his sleeves and do some-thing, anything. At the same time, seeing death as an everyday event makes one guilty and overly aware of one's own good fortune. As a field-worker, I was often made uncomfortable by what I saw. I felt I had stumbled into incredibly intimate and significant slices of patients' and doctors' lives. Much like any person who sees more than he would like of a friend's life, I felt guilty about some of the knowledge I had gained, worried over what the boundary between privileged information and data was, and wondered about how I repaid my obligation to my subjects. In the short run, the housestaff resolved the problem of helpless-ness and indebtedness by the roles they cast for me. When house-staff demanded that I help out by wheeling the chart rack, opening dressings, acting as a group memory, they provided me a means to cope with my own helplessness and assuage my guilt at the same time that they incorporated me into the group. While I was in the field, my involvement in the group resolved for me the problems I experienced as an indebted guest.

These problems reemerged when I left the field and began writing up the report. I saw much that was wrong in surgery, but what I saw emerged against the background of dedicated people working tirelessly at very difficult and complex tasks. What if what I reported was harmful to those that made the account possible? I had the problems of balancing my universal obligations to sociological analysis to my particular obligations to my research subjects. Unfortunately for me, I could not expect anyone to point the way by the everyday roles they cast me in. One thing I did was not begin writing immediately on leaving the field. Before drafting this report, I let the freshness of the experience recede somewhat so that I would not be overwhelmed by the memory of my relations with particular individuals. Second, when recording field notes, I made every attempt to keep my description of events as behavioral as possible, and my recording of conversations as verbatim as possible. At all times, I tried to keep "in situ" analysis separate from my field descriptions. I kept two different categories of field notes: (1) a log of happenings, conversations, and conferences; and (2) a separate running analysis. In this way I was later able to identify for and correct problems that resulted from overraport or over-indebtedness. By this procedure, I would see where the data confirmed, or failed to support, my analyses. There is in fieldwork always the problem of selective data collecting and analysis that might harm one's subjects. Any definitive resolution to this problem awaits more sophisticated, but at the same time unobtrusive, techniques of gathering field data. At the present, the length of time we spend in the field and our own intellectual integrity is our only protection to this problem. Third, I shared my report with the surgeons upon its completion. We discussed areas of disagreement between our interpretations. In particular, they objected to the rhetoric of sociology; they saw my framing the problem with a deviance and social-control vocabulary as unnecessarily pejorative, but they accepted (even if they did not

agree with or fully understand) my rationale. They agreed that I
had most of the phenomenological description right, if not always
the interpretations. However, where there were interpretive disagreements, the surgeons attributed them to my being a sociologist, and accepted my analysis as valid from my frame of reference. They suggested ways that I could better protect the
anonymity and confidentiality of individuals. For example, at
their request, I changed the pseudonyms I originally chose and
excised all dates from my field materials. I resolved part of my
debt by allowing the surgeons to observe me as a sociologist at
work.

Overgeneralization is also a recurrent problem for field-workers
at two levels. First, there is the danger that one particular event
will become etched in the field-worker's memory as emblematic of
the way action is organized in an environment. That is to say,
field-workers may overgeneralize incidents and see them as representative of categories of action. Second, field-workers may overgeneralize from their particular sites to all other types of similar
settings. In the first case, I avoided overgeneralization by making
sure I had at least two independently generated examples of
the same phenomenon before I began to make inferences. My
operating rule here was, as far as I can see, not fundamentally
different than those that survey researchers use to ensure reliability in their studies. Also, I was very careful to follow particular incidents through many levels of social organization. For
example, I was able to test my inferences about normative error in
the promotion meeting, where I observed the criteria attending
surgeons use to judge the fitness of housestaff for surgical careers.
Throughout my fieldwork, I was very careful to test observations
in one context against those of another. On the other hand, there
are observations I made that did not find their way into the
fieldwork because I felt my inferential base was too thin. On one
occasion I watched a series of unexpected deaths and complications, which occurred in quick succession, temporarily destroy
the morale of Able Service. These occurred during the end of a
rotation, while a chief resident was on vacation. I developed an
explanation which related the occurrence of failure and group

panic. However, during the rest of my fieldwork, I did not have the opportunity to observe another rash of failures. As a result, such speculations did not find their way into the manuscript. As an aid to the reader, I have tried to indicate throughout the text where inferences are based on slim observation.

There is a second type of overgeneralization—generalization from the specific case, Pacific Hospital, to hospitals that are not included in Pacific's class. Pacific is a member of the medical elite. There are perhaps twenty hospitals in this country with the same reputation for excellence that Pacific has. I am confident that the description of controls at Pacific is one that fits virtually all members of this class. I am also confident that I have described and analyzed a professional "ideal type," an environment where the major preoccupations have to do with the aesthetics and elegance of surgery, uncontaminated by such mundane matters as fees, social networks to generate referrals, and market pressures. How the system of social control I described is modified in more modal settings is a question that deserves further research, as is the question of how comparable it is to the systems of social control in other professions. These are questions that I am beginning to work on now. There is certainly no intrinsic reason that fieldwork cannot be as cumulative as any other area of sociology. The benefit of using a site like Pacific as a starting point is that physicians there are quite self-conscious about their place in the medical world, and make explicit reference to why they deserve an esteemed place in the profession. Moreover, being so self-conscious, they are eager to inculcate into their young recruits the values in which they believe so strongly. Attending surgeons see their trainees as extensions of themselves in many ways; one of these is that they expect the conduct of those whom they train to reflect honor and glory back on Pacific.

Out of the Field

One peculiarity of field research is that one discovers what one learns in the field often only after one has left the field. So, strangely, the most creative and fruitful periods of field research

are those where the researcher steps back from his immersion in
an alien world, takes stock, and decides where to go next. By
alternating periods of total immersion with periods of analysis,
the field-worker can avoid phenomenological fatigue, that is, the
sense of "I've seen it all before," and can continually refine and
sharpen the questions asked of a particular research. For this
study, I normally spent two or three months in the field, full-time,
recording my observations in as straightforward a manner as
possible, left the field for two weeks to a month to analyze my
data, and then returned with a greater sense of what I now knew
and what I still had to learn about the conduct of surgeons. For
example, after retreating from the field the first time, I discovered in my notes that surgeons treated some mistakes as
normal occurrences, while other events were treated as quite extraordinary and unacceptable performances. But at that time, I did
not know why one set of events was categorized by actors in one
way and another was so differently treated. It was clear very early
in the study that the seriousness of an error was not determined
by a set of precedent variables such as the patient's age or social
status, nor was it determined by such antecedent variables as
what happens to the patient. An error's seriousness was related
only incidentally to the patient and his condition. On the other
hand, seriousness was related in a very direct fashion to the
attending's reaction. Discovering this, I felt reassured and at the
same time I knew nothing, since I did not know what determined
the attending's reaction.

My first immersion in the field in some sense determined the
direction of most of my subsequent observation, as I tried to
unravel what the bases of attending evaluation were, how clear
these were to housestaff, and how widely they were shared among
all members of the team. A dialectic of immersion and reflection
that began the first day I arrived on the surgery wards at Pacific—
and which I am sure is not completed—allowed me a continuous
sense of discovery. It is worth noting, for instance, that I did not
discover quasi-normative errors until after I left the field entirely.
I had not seen while in the field so clearly how the lines of
cleavage among the ranks were structured. In turn, my new

understanding that there were two distinct types of normative error forced me to revise my conclusions about the social controls in surgical training by allowing me to see some of the ways its ethical content is undermined. I also gained a new respect for what it means "to let your field data speak to you." There are any number of things about the field that one discovers only by not being there. I discovered the "charisma" of surgery, not in the hospital but at parties and other social events. Being a sociologist does not normally make one the center of attention; however, being a sociologist who studies surgeons does. As my research progressed, I was struck by the almost primal awe my friends and acquaintances had for surgeons. Normally sophisticated urban dwellers with Simmel's (1970) blasé attitude would literally beg for details about what surgeons were really like, about what went on in operating rooms, about what their doctors were really like. It occurred to me that I had, through my close association with them, borrowed part of the surgeons' charisma. Seeing that the surgeons' charisma was not just some dramaturgic creation in organized social settings helped me understand how the surgeons' autonomy was as great and unchecked as it was. It also made me see that this was not simply a result of surgeons' behavior but was also nurtured by patients' needs and desires. Cocktail party curiosity also alerted me to how little people know about the medical care they receive, how few people have ever been in an operating room as an observer, and how powerful and coexistent are the contradictory impulses both to glorify and to degrade the surgeon. (Cocktail parties also taught me of the need for circumspection and tact, which I shall comment on below.)

Unfortunately, I did not learn as much from leaving the field as I might have, because I did not keep a careful record of why I chose to leave the field at the times I did. I assume that had I been as clear as I might about my comings and goings, about what was going on in the field that would make me willing or eager to leave, then I might have gained some greater understanding than I have about the surgeon's life space. I know there were days when I had to force myself to go to the hospital, and other days when I grabbed at any straw as an excuse for a breather. But when and why these feelings intensified at the times they did, I do not know. Such knowledge is of more than private psychodynamic interest (though it is of that also), for it helps make clear what strains field-workers are subject to in medical settings, how they can better prepare themselves, and how they can be better supervised. The end result from such understanding would be more valid and reliable monographs, less likely to be subject to any "observer effect."

Data, Confidentiality, and the Field-Worker

I indicated above that I learned some lessons at cocktail parties about circumspection. In a literal sense, this is not true; but social situations presented me with a sticky problem. When I was in the middle of the field, disguising the place and principals of my study was not as easy as it is in this report. I was always aware when I spoke that others knew those I spoke of, and that a too-loose tongue could hurt me and them in many untold ways. Since I promised my subjects confidentiality and anonymity, the "cover story" I devised to manage social situations was as consequential as the one I devised to manage field introductions. Only by assuring confidentiality and anonymity could I satisfy my subjects that my study would be within the bounds of current medical ethics. Both promises present some dilemmas, however.

First, I could not ever be sure that some enterprising person would not be able to figure out my place and principals. Essentially, confidentiality and anonymity were the promises I made but I had little control over their fulfillment. There have been recent debates about whether field-workers should go to the bother of making general "covering names" for their sites, and whether they should disguise their subjects. It seems to me that such fictitious names do more than provide confidentiality and anonymity: they highlight the generalized features of our descriptions and minimize the particularized aspects. To my mind, this aspect of naming is even more important in some ways than confidentiality and anonymity in that it creates a fieldwork literature rather than a description of specific places; for example, Bellevue, Long Island Jewish Hospital, Johns Hopkins.

Others have advocated that to make fieldwork more rigorous and to display our methodology more openly, we should open our notebooks to the curious. Such procedure would allow others to see how we manipulate our data and fit the canons of science in general. Such a proposal troubles me because, as a sociologist, I gathered litigable material from subjects who trusted me. As a sociologist, I have no legal right to claim a privileged or confidential relationship with my subjects; my notes are subpoenable. If I opened my notebooks in the manner necessary to make clear the operations I performed on my data, I risk having those notebooks put to uses other than those I approve of by people whose motives I may distrust for reasons I think are less than just. Involved here is a difficult problem: how to afford my subjects and myself enough protection so that we feel comfortable doing the study, at the same time displaying my data in a way that assures others of the validity and reliability of my research. I have indicated for the reader what I have done to satisfy myself of this report's accuracy. For the moment, I suggest that this—along with giving and receiving adequate supervision—is the best I can do.

Conclusion

As a research method, fieldwork yields results that often are phenomenologically rich, theoretically provocative, and practically useful. The major liability with this research method is that there are no procedures internal to the techniques of field research itself that control validity and reliability. The major data-gathering technique that the researcher utilizes is his relationship with his subjects. For better or worse the rules that govern relationships are less precise, harder to articulate, and more complexly interwoven with other normative systems than the rules that govern, for example, item construction on a questionnaire. By the same token, the field-worker's sampling procedures and

the manipulations he performs on his data are often left unex-
plained. Clearly it is not that field-workers do not gather data by
rules, sample from everyday life in a complex fashion, or manipulate their data. Rather, it is the case that to state what the rules are
requires statements of such generality that they are of little use
in any particular setting. The reason for this is not hard to understand: our subjects are never simply subjects. They also occupy a
variety of other roles and the rules that govern relationships, for
example, with physicians are different than those that govern
relationships with heroin addicts. This inherent variation imposes
on the field-worker his special obligation. The field-worker must
describe the role relations that he had with his subjects as clearly
and honestly as he can. The field-worker must describe how he
avoided overinvolvement or on what occasions he succumbed to
it, how he avoided overgeneralizing, and how he avoided overindebtedness to his subjects. A clear statement of the social
matrix out of which the field materials emerged allows the reader
to judge validity and reliability for himself. At the same time, it
has the added benefit of providing comparable accounts of the
fieldwork experience which allows us to see what is general to a
researcher's relations to his subject and what is particularly his
own.

Notes

Chapter Two

1. The sociological literature on accounts and motives deals with breached expectations. Worthy of special note are Dewey (1922); Lyman and Scott (1968); Foote (1951); Blum and McHugh (1971); and Mills (1944).

2. An acceptable answer in everyday terms is one which renders further questions unnecessary. It ends the search procedure. (See Churchill 1971.)

3. Orderly surgical activity occurs when attending surgeons have their plans carried out with little disruption by deaths and complications—physiological accident—or by others in the work group—social accident.

4. Citations with a name indicate interview material. Citations with service indicate participant-observer data.

5. I am grateful to Edward Shils (1975) for the conceptual imagery. Recently Barber et al. (1973) have questioned Merton's (1957) conception of medical schools as moral leaders. Right or wrong, Barber and his colleagues are somewhat beside the point. Medical schools, as they suggest, may not provide much in the way of moral leadership, but they are the only leadership the next generation of physicians has.

6. See chapter 7.

7. Two good early discussions of uncertainty are Fox (1957) and Davis (1960). Fox discusses how physicians learn to manage uncertainty as students; Davis deals with its control implications in the doctor-patient relationship.

Chapter Three

1. The traffic of rounds provides interesting grist for two of Goffman's mills: vehicular traffic (1971) and deference patterns (1967).

2. Freidson (1970a) discusses these in a different context.

3. Here it is perhaps necessary to remind the reader that a distinctive feature of surgical training is that until one reaches attending status the

direct orders of superordinates are seen as legitimate (see Goss 1961; Stelling and Bucher 1972; and Miller 1970).

4. There is a rich underground lore among surgeons about researchers whose procedures were less than scientific.

5. The distinction between board-certified and occasional surgeons becomes meaningful given the great amount of surgery done by noncertified surgeons in this country. The board-certified surgeons claim that this is a major flaw in our delivery system: they cannot control surgery unless they can control who may act as surgeons. The power to decide who may do surgery is currently in the hands of hospital trustees who are often members of religious or fraternal orders; rarely are they professionals. A few times when I asked Arthur about controls at hospitals other than Pacific, he answered: "Five pounds of candy to Mother Superior at Christmastime will cover a multitude of sins." By which I suppose he meant to make perfectly clear the nonprofessional manner in which work in a hospital is regulated.

Chapter Four

1. Field researchers (see Dalton 1959) have noted this phenomenon— the loose-mouthedness of the malcontent—as a general problem in coding the reliability of information that their field subjects pass on to them. Undoubtedly members of an organization are as aware as field researchers of this, but how they weight information against its source in building up their own interpretation of what is "really" going on is a largely unexplored topic.

2. As subordinates who must account for failure to superordinates are well aware, one person's backstage is another's center. Backstage refers to spaces where actors may retreat and allow some distance between themselves and their roles. I would speculate that the relationship between backstage privacy and status is U-shaped. The very poor, those who command no social resources, cannot afford a backstage area; and the very celebrated are often followed far backstage: Bob Dylan and Henry Kissinger's garbage is ransacked. Jacqueline Onassis and Photographer Ray Gaella bickered in court for quite some time over when public curiosity invades private backstage and becomes a public nuisance. Recently, how far televised news may invade the private spaces of private individuals during public disasters has become a question of journalistic ethics (see *New York Times*, 6 July 1975, Arts and Leisure Section, p. 1).

3. The background resources that participants employ for under-standing such action literally without thinking is the basic problem that ethnomethodology explores. Garfinkel (1967) and his followers (Sudnow [1972] is an especially useful collection) have demonstrated how much work sustains the most ordinary interactions. Such work demonstrates how problematic cell 1 can be when subject to scrutiny. However, I have noticed that the field-workers who take Garfinkel's ideas seriously pay little heed to his chief methodological injunction: "Procedurally, it is my preference to start with familiar scenes and ask what can be done to produce trouble. The operations that one would have to perform in order to multiply the senseless features of the perceived environments to pro-duce and sustain bewilderment, consternation, and confusion; to pro-duce the socially structured effects of anxiety, shame and guilt, and indignation; and to produce disorganized interaction should say some-thing about how the structures of everyday activity are ordinarily produced and maintained" (pp. 37–38). Field-researchers of an ethno-methodological frame of mind do not go out and create troubles—this is reserved for experimentalists (see McHugh 1968)—rather, they ask what participants in a scene see as their normal troubles and how they manage them to create artful interactions (for good examples, see Bittner 1967; Sudnow 1965, 1967; and Emerson 1970). There is in this approach a convergence with Hughes' suggestions for studying occupa-tions and the world of work.

4. Two features of the medical environment are important in under-standing why such questioning occurs as it does. First, there is the depth of the student's unfamiliarity with surgery. The students I observed almost uniformly expressed their surprise at the following: that immed-iately following surgery, previously healthy-looking individuals appeared so sick. Attendings work on convincing them that this is "normal" and "no cause for alarm." Here a few good results go a long way in refocus-ing student concern from patient-oriented to procedure-oriented con-cerns, that is, from worrying about an individual bleeding to the methods used to control bleeding. Second, there is the surgeon's sensi-tivity to the stereotype other specialists hold of him as a mere "tinkerer," a "technician," or a "body plumber." Attendings and residents are well aware of and resent these views. As a result, surgeons spend a great deal of their time demonstrating to students the sophistication of their clinical reasoning. Undoubtedly some of this is encouraged by the academic climate; however, some of it appears as defensive reaction to a negative stereotype.

5. Two digressions are in order here. First, much of the surgery in medical potboilers and television dramas seems to be of this sort. In everyday life, when such dramatic surgery succeeds, it is often considered highly newsworthy, especially when the beneficiaries are young children. I suspect that if one were to take an index of articles in popular media about modern medical miracles, a greater proportion than one would expect by chance would be about pediatric patients—an indicator of how highly this society values youth.

Second, a question that I quite consistently and consciously bracketed during my field research was whether surgeons had met the demands of ethics and the law and obtained the "informed consent" of those patients for whom they wished to work miracles. I did not suspend judgment because I considered this problem unimportant. Quite to the contrary, it is one of the most complex and consequential questions one can ask about the delivery of care and the nature of professional-client relationships. I suspended judgment and bracketed the question because I was interested in surgeons' understandings of their social control responsibilities and in their definitions of error and failure. Whether the demands of "informed consent" were met or not was not a matter that surgeons considered a matter for social control. The quality of the consent obtained is not an issue that excites surgeons or affects their evaluation of each other. Moreover, I felt that acting as a conscience for my subjects and reminding them that "informed consent" was a matter that they should police would have been inappropriate; it would have made me a participant-advocate instead of a participant-observer.

I think that it is a sad commentary that in order to enter into the everyday world of surgeons one has to bracket such questions. However, it is also not clear whether a consideration of such matters would make surgeons any better or worse as surgeons. Here I apply the surgeon's own criteria of quality, which are clinical and narrow. Moreover, we might not be surprised that if the attending surgeon does not share his deliberations with his subordinates, he will not feel obligated to share them with his patients.

Further, there is in the very notion of "informed consent" as its definition has evolved a paradox that makes its achievement a virtual impossibility. To wit, to satisfy the demands of "informed consent," a surgeon, any physician, must, when suggesting a treatment to a patient, inform him of alternative treatments and their risks and benefits as compared to the proposed treatment. The patient's consent to treatment should ideally be free and not coerced. However, when the physician presents alternatives to the patient, he himself has already been persuaded of which alternative he prefers. So persuaded, it is hard to imagine that when he lays out to the patient his options, the physician does not order his discussion as a convincing argument for the alternative he favors and coerce the patient by his own belief in the correctness of his judgment. Hard to imagine because this is the way he has been taught to discourse on medical problems since his own training began.

In medicine, as opposed to sociology, making a diagnosis is not a value-free activity. Diagnosis is the rationale for intervention. It commits one to a course of action. Clinicians cannot leave the policy implications of their diagnoses for others to worry over. This is a luxury of sociologists and not of physicians in general or surgeons in particular.

Now, if the patient is informed of treatment plans by the physician's argument for what he thinks should be done, it is hard to conceive of truly informed consent for arguments themselves are structured by emphasizing some facts, minimizing some facts, and neglecting others entirely. If this is so, the physician's mode of discussion prevents him from laying out options in the impartial manner informed consent requires. Further, were he to do so, he might undermine the patient's trust and faith in his magical powers to cure—a trust and faith that medical anthropology informs us is an important part of the cure itself (Levi-Strauss 1963).

6. Unfortunately, I do not have data on the distribution of cases at Grand Rounds for the period of this study. However, the chief resident responsible for organizing the conference frequently voiced his concern to me that no service be underrepresented or overrepresented.

7. In the early days of open-heart surgery, there developed an interesting phenomenon known as the "Lazarus" syndrome, which is a corollary to patient presentation at rounds. Here, the surgeon waits in the recovery room with the patient and as he is coming out of anesthesia whispers in his ear: "You're alive. You're alive" (personal communication from David Schneider, Ph.D.). The syndrome is named for Lazarus rather than Christ, I imagine, more for the intensity of a patient's fear surrounding surgery, the awareness of the once-stopped heart beating again, and the patient's feeling that he has literally been raised from the dead than for the innate modesty and sense of propriety of cardiac surgeons. Patient presentation at Grand Rounds serves as evidence that all attendings have their Lazaruses and hence their opportunities to play Christ.

8. Coser (1961) and Hughes (1971) provide nice statements on how

guilty knowledge is shared by superordinates and subordinates. For all
the protection attendings afford housestaff, they are given a great deal in
return. In fact, a great danger to the professional whose activities are
invisible to all but a handful of trusted subordinates is that a sharer of
guilty knowledge will go public (see "Nurses Trigger Doctor Quiz,"
Chicago Tribune, 28 August 1974, p. 1). The codes of silence as they
exist within licit and illicit occupations (see Maas 1968; Talese 1971) are
a very revealing aspect of group life. The secret has received little
attention since Simmel and deserves a great deal more. What people
choose and work to keep unknown says much about them. The fit
between the skeletons and the clothes in the closet is always of some
interest and importance.

9. The retrospective peer-review conference conducted by the Department of Surgery differs considerably from the one conducted by the
Department of Internal Medicine. In this latter conference, only one or
two cases of interest are reported on. They are chosen for their heuristic
value. They are intensively researched. Their presentation is separated
from their occurrence by six to eight weeks. There is no attempt at this
conference or elsewhere to make public and demand accounts for each
death and complication that occurs as there is in the surgical conference.
The public accounting of surgeons also differs considerably from what
Light (1972) reports for psychiatrists.

Thus far, the literature on peer review has concentrated on the prospective review of clinical research (Gray 1975; Barber et al. 1973). These
researchers conclude that such review improves the ethical performance
of researchers, but how great such improvement is remains difficult to
measure. The same problems exist for measuring the effectiveness of
retrospective peer review. When questioned, all housestaff reported that
one could and that they indeed did learn from the Mortality and Morbidity Conference. However, at the same time, they also expressed the
belief that the best way to learn to manage complications was by actually managing them—an echo of the surgery-as-a-body-contact-sport
philosophy.

10. This rule has an elastic quality about it; namely, the more minor
the complication and the more happy the outcome, the more likely that
the complication will be seen as "just one of those things," and the more
likely that the subordinate will have complete accounting responsibility.
In such cases the subordinate's original accounting to the attending is a
dramatic rehearsal of the explanation he must later give in public.

11. An interesting feature of the presentation of such cases is that the recitation of a long list of injuries indicating a hopeless situation provokes anxious laughter among members of the audience.

12. The attending is obliged only by his own sense of his role and mission; he need not step forward, he may allow his subordinate to take the heat or he may absent himself entirely from the conference. Such a course of action is fraught with danger for attendings, however. I will discuss these dangers below.

13. The dynamics by which authority is undermined fall outside the already broad scope of this study. My impressions as far as attendings are concerned are sketchy since I was not so much an insider among them that attendings carried tales to me of each other's behavior. As far as subordinates are concerned, my impressions rest on a firmer basis. The housestaff on Baker accepted Arthur's authority despite his histrionics because they respected his integrity—it was a popular topic of conversation. On Able, where White and Peters were less open, authority was more subject to breakdown.

14. The concern with impression-management and saving face (Goffman 1967) has perhaps blinded us to the dynamics of altruistic sacrifice of face.

Chapter Five

1. This is not to say that no controls exist beyond this point but rather that this is the last institutionally structured one. Superordinates can drum offensive subordinates out of training at any point. However, the longer training continues, the greater is the burden of proof required to discredit an individual and thereby oust him. Second, the institutionalization of decision making can soften the blow for those who do not make the grade. The claim can legitimately be made that the decision is no reflection on them but testimony to how stiff the competition was that year. So, as a general rule, the longer one continues to train beyond the institutionalized decision-making point, the more difficult it is to separate him from the training program. This is a case of "If it were done when 'tis done, then 'twere well / It were done quickly" (*Macbeth*, act 1, scene 7).

2. Freidson and Rhea (1972) identify exclusion as the primary social control mechanism in a group practice. Freidson, in other writings (1970), identifies exclusion as the primary social control mechanism of

the medical profession. I extend these earlier discussions by showing the logic that physicians apply in deciding whom to exclude and whom to include.

3. Miller (1970) has borrowed Matza's (1964) concept of drift to explain the careers of interns in an elite training program. The term seems inappropriate for two reasons. First, a career in an elite institution requires the commitment of too much time and energy to be unthinkingly pursued. Second, superordinates play a too-important role in determining the currents subordinates are allowed to drift within. I think that in his interpretation Miller mistook what might have been a defensive rationalization subordinates used to soothe failure for a social process. Presumably people experience a great deal more difficulty than cream in drifting to the top.

4. Moreover, I suspect from my observations, but lack systematic evidence, that it is normative compliance rather than technical proficiency which leads attendings to choose subordinates as assistants on research. I expect a positive relationship between normative skills and sponsorship.

Chapter Six

1. Young physicians are taught techniques that encourage the patient to think he is "special" to the physician—always sit when visiting patients in their rooms, escort them from your clinic personally, develop a theme from their lives and structure discussion around it.

2. Retractors are known in the argot of surgery as "idiotsticks." The phrase conveys the degree of skill necessary to hold them properly. The maintenance of interest while standing at attention and keeping the patient's flesh clear of the operative field for hours on end is no easy task. However, superordinates take an inability to do this as an indication that an individual does not care about becoming a surgeon. Further, flagging interest insults the attending who is operating: he expects that his art will be appreciated for art's sake, if not merely for the utilitarian lessons a subordinate may learn.

Bibliography

Barber, Bernard; Lally, John J.; Makarushka, Julia Loughlin; and Sullivan, Daniel. *Research on Human Subjects: Problems of Social Control in Medical Experimentation.* New York: Russell Sage, 1973.

Becker, Howard. *Outsiders: Studies in the Sociology of Deviance.* New York: Free Press, 1963.

———. *Sociological Work: Method and Substance.* Chicago: Aldine, 1970.

Becker, Howard; Geer, Blanche; Hughes, Everett C.; and Strauss, Anselm. *Boys in White: Student Culture in Medical School.* Chicago: University of Chicago Press, 1961.

Bensman, Joseph, and Gerver, Israel. "Crime and Punishment in the Factory: The Function of Deviancy in Maintaining a Social System." *American Sociological Review* 28(1963):588-99.

Bittner, Egon. "The Police on Skid Row." *American Sociological Review* 32(1967a):239-58.

———. "Police Discretion in the Apprehension of Mentally Ill Persons." *Social Problems* 14(1967b):278-92.

Blum, Alan, and McHugh, Peter. "The Social Ascription of Motives." *American Sociological Review* 31(1971):98-109.

Bossert, Steven. "Tasks and Social Relationships in the Classroom." Ph.D. dissertation, University of Chicago, 1975.

Bucher, Rue. "Conflicts and Transformations of Identity: A Study of Medical Specialists." Ph.D. dissertation, University of Chicago, 1961.

Bucher, Rue, and Strauss, Anselm. "Professions in Process." *American Journal of Sociology* 66(1961):325-34.

Churchill, Lindsay. "Ethnomethodology and Measurement." *Social Forces* 50(1971):182-91.

Cicourel, Aaron. *The Social Organization of Juvenile Justice.*
New York: Wiley, 1969.

Cook, Robin. *The Year of the Intern.* New York: Signet Books,
1972.

Coser, Rose Laub. "Authority and Decision-Making in a Hospital." *American Sociological Review* 23(1958):56–63.

———. "Insulation from Observability and Types of Social
Control." *American Sociological Review* 26(1961):28–39.

Crane, Diana. *The Sanctity of Social Life.* New York: Russell
Sage, 1975.

Dalton, Melville. *Men Who Manage.* New York: John Wiley,
1959.

Daniels, Arlene K. "Military Psychiatry: The Emergence of a
Sub-specialty." In *Medical Men and Their Work*, edited by
Eliot Freidson and Judith Lorber. Chicago: Aldine-Atherton,
1972, pp. 145–62.

Daniels, Morris. "Affect and its Control in the Intern." *American Journal of Sociology* 66(1961):259–67.

Davis, Fred. "Uncertainty in Medical Diagnosis: Clinical and
Functional." *American Journal of Sociology* 66(1960):41–47.

Dewey, John. *Human Nature and Conduct.* New York: Modern
Library, 1922.

Emerson, Joan. "Behavior in Private Places: Sustaining Definitions of Reality in Gynecological Exams." In *Recent Sociology,
No. 2,* edited by Hans Dreitzel. New York: Macmillan, 1970,
pp. 73–97.

Erikson, K. T. *Wayward Puritans.* New York: John Wiley: 1966.

Foote, Nelson. "Identification as the Basis for a Theory of Motivation." *American Sociological Review* 16(1951):14–21.

Fox, Renée C. "Training for Uncertainty." In *The Student-Physician,* edited by Robert K. Merton, George Reader, and Patricia
Kendall. Cambridge: Harvard University Press, 1957*a*, pp.
207–41.

———. "The Autopsy: Its Place in the Attitude-Learning of
Second-Year Medical Students." Department of Sociology,
University of Pennsylvania, 1957*b*, unpublished.

———. *Experiment Perilous.* New York: Free Press, 1959.

—————. "Ethical and Existential Developments in Contemporaneous American Medicine: Their Implications for Culture and Society." *Millbank Memorial Fund Quarterly*, Fall 1974, pp. 445-83.

Fox, Renée C., and Lief, Harold. "Training for 'Detached Concern' in Medical Students." In *The Psychological Basis of Medical Practice*, edited by Harold Lief, Victor Lief, and Nina Lief. New York: Harper and Row, 1963, pp. 12-35.

Freidson, Eliot. "Client Control and Medical Practice." *American Journal of Sociology* 65(1960):374-82.

—————. *The Profession of Medicine: A Study in the Sociology of Applied Knowledge.* New York: Harper and Row, 1970*a*.

—————. *Professional Dominance: The Social Structure of Medical Care.* New York: Atherton, 1970*b*.

—————. *Doctoring Together.* New York: Elsevier, 1975.

Freidson, Eliot, and Rhea, Buford. "Processes of Control in a Company of Equals." In *Medical Men and Their Work*, edited by Eliot Freidson and Judith Lorber. Chicago: Aldine-Atherton, 1972, pp. 185-89.

Garfinkel, Harold. "Conditions of Successful Degradation Ceremonies." *American Journal of Sociology* 61(1956):420-24.

—————. *Studies in Ethnomethodology.* Englewood Cliffs, N.J.: Prentice-Hall, 1967.

Glaser, Barney, and Strauss, Anselm. *The Discovery of Grounded Theory: Strategies for Qualitative Research.* Chicago: Aldine, 1967.

Glaser, Ronald J. *Ward 402.* New York: Braziller, 1973.

Goffman, Erving. *The Presentation of Self in Everyday Life.* Garden City, N.J.: Anchor-Doubleday, 1959.

—————. *Encounters: Two Studies in the Sociology of Interaction.* Indianapolis: Bobbs-Merrill, 1961.

—————. *Interaction Ritual: Essays on Face-to-Face Behavior.* Garden City, N.J.: Anchor-Doubleday, 1967.

—————. *Relations in Public.* New York: Harper, 1971.

Goode, W. J. "Protection of the Inept." *American Sociological Review* 32(1967):5-19.

Goss, Mary E. W. "Influence and Authority among Physicians in an Outpatient Clinic." *American Sociological Review* 26(1961): 39-50.

Gray, Bradford H. *Human Subjects in Medical Experimentation.* New York: John Wiley, 1975.

Halberstam, David. *The Best and the Brightest.* New York: Fawcett, 1972.

Hughes, Everett C. *The Sociological Eye: Selected Papers on Work, Self, and Society.* Chicago: Aldine-Atherton, 1971.

Icheiser, Gustav. *Appearances and Realities.* San Francisco: Jossey-Bass, 1972.

Janowitz, Morris. *Social Control of the Welfare State.* Chicago: University of Chicago Press, 1976.

Levi-Strauss, Claude. *Structural Anthropology.* New York: Basic Books, 1963.

Lidz, Charles. "Rethinking Rapport: Problems of Reciprocal Obligations in Participant Observation Research." Paper presented at the annual meeting of the Eastern Sociological Association. New York, March 1977.

Light, Donald. "Psychiatry and Suicide: The Management of a Mistake." *American Journal of Sociology* 77(1972):821-38.

———. "The Sociological Calendar: An Analytic Tool." *American Journal of Sociology* 80(1975):1145-64.

Lukes, Steven. *Essays in Social Theory.* New York: Columbia University Press, 1977.

Lyman, Stanford, and Scott, Marvin. "Accounts." *American Sociological Review* 33(1968):46-62.

Maas, Peter. *The Valachi Papers.* New York: Putnam, 1968.

McHugh, Peter. *Defining the Situation.* Indianapolis: Bobbs-Merrill Co., 1968.

Matza, David. *Delinquency and Drift.* New York: John Wiley, 1964.

Mauss, Marcel. *The Gift.* New York: W. W. Norton, 1967.

Merton, Robert K. "Some Preliminaries to a Sociology of Medical Education." In *The Student-Physician*, edited by Robert K. Merton, George Reader, and Patricia Kendall. Cambridge: Harvard University Press, 1957, pp. 3-81.

Miller, Steven J. *Prescription for Leadership: Training for the Medical Elite.* Chicago: Aldine, 1970.

Mills, C. Wright. "Situated Actions and a Vocabulary of Mo-
tives." *American Sociological Review* 5(1944):904-13.
Mumford, Emily. *Interns: From Students to Physicians.* Cam-
bridge: Harvard University Press, 1970.
Nolen, William J. *The Making of a Surgeon.* New York: Random
House, 1970.
————. *A Surgeon's World.* New York: Random House, 1972.
Parsons, Talcott. *Essays in Sociological Theory.* New York: Free
Press, 1949.
————. *The Social System.* New York: Free Press, 1951.
————. "Professions." In *The International Encyclopedia of the
Social Sciences.* New York: Macmillan, 1968, pp. 536-47.
Schwartz, Barry. "Waiting, Power, and Exchange: The Distribu-
tion of Time in Social Systems." *American Journal of Socio-
logy* 79(1974):841-71.
Shils, Edward. *Center and Periphery: Essays in Macrosociology.*
Chicago: University of Chicago Press, 1975.
Siegler, Mark. "Pascal's Wager and the Hanging of Crepe." *New
England Journal of Medicine* 293(1975):853-57.
Simmel, Georg. *On Individuality and Social Forms,* edited by
Donald Levine. Chicago: University of Chicago Press, 1970.
Smelser, Neil J. *Theory of Collective Behavior.* London: Rout-
ledge & Kegan Paul, 1962.
Stelling, Joan, and Bucher, Rue. "Autonomy and Monitoring on
Hospital Wards." *Sociological Quarterly* 13(1972):431-47.
Sudnow, David. "Normal Crimes." *Social Problems* 12(1965):
255-76.
————. *Passing On: The Social Organization of Dying.* Engle-
wood Cliffs, N.J.: Prentice-Hall, 1967.
————, ed. *Studies in Interaction.* New York: Free Press, 1972.
Sykes, Gresham, and Matza, David. "Techniques of Neutraliza-
tion: A Theory of Delinquency." *American Sociological Review*
22(1957):667-69.
Talese, Gay. *Honor Thy Father.* New York: World Publishers,
1971.
Viscott, David J. *The Making of a Psychiatrist.* New York: Arbor
House, 1974.
Webb, Eugene; Campbell, D. T.; Schwartz, R. D.; and Sechrest,

L. *Unobtrusive Measures: Nonreactive Research in the Social Sciences.* Chicago: Rand McNally, 1966.

Wender, Paul. "Vicious and Virtuous Circles: The Role of Deviation-Amplifying Feedback in the Origin and Perpetuation of Behavior." *Psychiatry* 31(1968):309–24.

X, Dr. *Intern.* New York: Harper and Row, 1965.

Zimmerman, Donald. "The Practicalities of Rule Use." In *Understanding Everyday Life,* edited by Jack Douglas. Chicago: Aldine, 1970, pp. 221–38.

Index

Able service, 8–11, 32, 69, 99, 103–4,
109, 197; attendings on, 10–11, 79,
81; authority on, 221; errors on, 13,
38–39, 41–42, 45–47, 52–54, 64;
exogenous failure on, 69; help
seeking on, 44; morale on, 207,
208; Mortality and Morbidity Conferences on, 145, 146; research
orientation of, 10, 11
Access to site, 194, 195
Accounts, 5, 31, 36, 98, 114, 215, 220;
and attendings, 96–97, 112–14;
relativity of, 30; responsibility and,
49, 50; strategies of, 129–30, 135–
36; and surgery, 30; types of, 141,
142; unnecessary, 120, 121. *See
also* Responsibility
Altruism, 221
American College of Surgeons, 58
Anesthesiologists, 105
Anonymity, 211, 212
Atherton, Bruce, x
Attendings, 3, 8–9, 11, 90, 123–24; and
accounts, 96–97, 113–14; as arbitrary, 89, 146; authority of, 84–86,
92, 113, 216; and competition, 150;
and conferences, 221; disagreements between, 9; discipline by, 84,
161; excuses and, 57–58, 76, 97–
98, 100; and fieldworker, 193–94,
197–98, 200–201; gatekeeping
function of, 148, 149; and housestaff, 37–38, 84; and judgmental
errors, 45, 48–49, 112; in Mortality
and Morbidity Conferences, 134–
36, 146; and normative errors,

53–55, 57–60; and quasi-normative
errors, 61–67; and residents, 158,
159; rounds of, 11–12, 79–84; and
students, 217; and technical errors,
37, 39, 112
Authority, 61, 201; attendings and,
84–86, 92; breakdown of, 221;
levels of, 9, 10; medical, 85; respect
for, 59; and scientific evidence, 86,
87; surgical, 65; undermining of,
221; Weber on, 113
Autonomy, zones of, 82
Autopsies, 174

Backstage, 112, 113; relativity of, 216
Baker service, 12–13, 32, 89, 91–94,
99–102, 105, 107, 109; attendings
on, 12–13, 79, 81, 83; chart rounds
on, 78; clinical experience on, 87,
88; decision making on, 96; expected failure on, 119, 120; Grand
Rounds on, 126, 127; judgmental
errors on, 49; Mortality and Morbidity Conferences on, 136–37,
145; normative errors on, 54–55,
59–60; quasi-normative errors on,
62–65, 67; scientific evidence
on, 86–89; technical errors on, 42–
43; work rounds on, 76
"Bandits," 187, 188
Barber, Bernard, 21, 188, 190, 215,
220, 223
Beatings, 6
Becker, Howard, 19–20, 205, 223
Bensman, Joseph, 223
Bershady, Harold, ix